Dear Susan

Dear Susan

*Letters of Comfort, Hope, and Peace for
Women Facing a Life-Changing Illness*

Ronda Barney, LCSW, RD

Library of Congress Control Number: 2021923208

Softcover: 978-1-64746-962-7
Hardcover: 978-1-64746-963-4
E-book: 978-1-64746-964-1

Available in hardcover, softcover, e-book, and audiobook.

All Scripture quotations marked (NIV) are taken from the Holy Bible, New
International Version®, NIV®. Copyright © 1973, 1978, 1984, 2011 by Biblica,
Inc.™ Used by permission of Zondervan. All rights reserved worldwide. www.
zondervan.com The"NIV" and "New International Version" are trademarks
registered in the United States Patent and Trademark Office by Biblica, Inc.™

Scripture quotations taken from the (NASB®) New American Standard Bible®,
Copyright © 1960, 1971, 1977, 1995, 2020, by The Lockman Foundation.
Used by permission. All rights reserved. www.lockman.org

Scripture quotations marked (AMP) are taken from the Amplified Bible,
Copyright © 2015 by The Lockman Foundation. Used by permission.

Scripture quotations marked (ESV) are taken from The Holy Bible, English
Standard Version® (ESV®) Copyright © 2001 by Crossway, a publishing
ministry of Good News Publishers. All rights reserved.

Scripture quotations noted (NKJV) are taken from the New King James
Version®. Copyright ©1982 by Thomas Nelson. Used by permission.
All rights reserved.

The information provided in this book is for informational purposes only.
This book is not intended to be or to substitute for medical advice, and
it should not be used to diagnose or treat an illness. Readers should
consult with their personal healthcare practitioners before implementing
suggestions or inferences from this book. The author and publisher expressly
disclaim responsibility for any adverse effects from the use of information
contained in this book. All healthcare decisions should be made in
conjunction with advice from a qualified healthcare professional.

Any Internet addresses provided in this book are offered as a resource.
They are not intended in any way to be or imply an endorsement by Author
Academy Elite, nor does Author Academy Elite or Ronda Barney vouch for
the content of these sites for the life of this book.

This book is dedicated to my dear husband, Chris, my two grown treasured kids, Seth and Raegan, the posse of friends who have walked this road with me, and my precious friend, Susan.

Each of you has given me the gifts of unconditional love, patience, and grace. Without you, this book would not be possible.

CONTENTS

FOREWORD xiii

A NOTE TO CAREGIVERS,
    FAMILY, AND FRIENDS xvii

A NOTE TO THE READER xix

LET ME INTRODUCE MYSELF xxiii

LETTERS TO SUSAN

THE STORY OF MY HEART. 1
    JOURNAL. 4

YOU ARE NOT A BURDEN 5
    JOURNAL. 7

DO YOU FEEL INVISIBLE?. 8
    JOURNAL. 11

IT'S OK TO GRIEVE 12
    JOURNAL. 14

HERE'S A RED RIBBON OF HOPE. . . . 15
    JOURNAL. 17

THE TRUTH ABOUT FAILURE 18
    JOURNAL. 21

TIRED OF THE FEAR 22
    JOURNAL. 24

MOVING FROM FROZEN TO FORWARD. . 25
    JOURNAL. 27

THIS IS NOT PUNISHMENT. 28
    JOURNAL. 31

LET ME TELL YOU
    MY GREATEST FEAR. 32
    JOURNAL. 35

AWAKEN TO HOPE 36
    JOURNAL. 39

THE MIND-BODY CONNECTION 40
    JOURNAL. 43

ISOLATED BUT NOT ALONE 44
    JOURNAL. 46

LET'S DANCE 47
    JOURNAL. 50

EMBRACING UNCONDITIONAL LOVE. . 51
    JOURNAL. 54

SETBACKS ARE SO HARD 55
    JOURNAL. 57

CAN YOU DO THIS MOMENT?. 58
    JOURNAL. 61

JOY, AN INSIDE JOB 62
    JOURNAL. 65

THE VALUE OF REST 66
    JOURNAL. 69

MY GREAT REWARD 70
   JOURNAL. 72

ANOTHER SETBACK 73
   JOURNAL. 75

THE POWER OF CHOICE 76
   JOURNAL. 79

THE STING OF TERMINAL 80
   JOURNAL. 82

IN THE WAITING. 83
   JOURNAL. 85

YOU MATTER 86
   JOURNAL. 88

YOUR BODY IS FOR YOU 89
   JOURNAL. 92

WHAT DOES THE WORD
"SURRENDER" MEAN TO YOU? . . . 93
   JOURNAL. 98

TRYING TO GET "HER" BACK 99
   JOURNAL. .102

THERE IS GOOD. 103
   JOURNAL. .105

THE OPPORTUNITY OF
VULNERABILITY 106
   JOURNAL. .108

DEVELOPING CLEARER VISION 109
   JOURNAL. .112

DO YOU FEEL FORGOTTEN?. 113
   JOURNAL. 115

THE STORY YOU TELL YOURSELF 116
   JOURNAL. 118

I GET TO TAKE CARE OF ME. 119
   JOURNAL. 122

GRATITUDE 123
   JOURNAL. 125

LIVING A LIFE OF ABUNDANCE. 126
   JOURNAL. 129

HOPE, FAITH & LOVE 130
   JOURNAL. 133

LONGING TO LIVE PAIN-FREE. 134
   JOURNAL. 138

LEARNING TO SOAR 139
   JOURNAL. 142

APPENDICES

LET'S KEEP IN TOUCH. 143

IN MEMORIAM OF SUSAN C. NEIBEL. .145

THANK YOU LETTER 147

ABOUT THE AUTHOR. 149

FOREWORD

I have stage 4 terminal cancer and am now receiving hospice care. The first time the doctors diagnosed and successfully treated the cancer was in 2007. Unfortunately, in 2018, it returned with a more severe prognosis requiring new, intense treatments.

Despite having insight into the medical system acquired over many years as an ICU nurse, supplemented by being blessed with loving family and friends, my knowledge and their support were insufficient. Unprepared for the emotional roller coaster of ups and downs that often accompany treatment for an incurable illness, I needed someone who had walked in my shoes to help me cope with the trauma that comes when hope is crushed by harsh reality.

In June 2020, I met Ronda Barney. I didn't realize at the time how significant that introduction would become but quickly discovered she came along at just the right time. Ronda had already begun writing this book of letters to encourage individuals going through difficulties similar to what she had experienced and felt led by God to address each letter with the salutation, "Dear Susan".

Ronda began writing in 2018, just two months prior to my second diagnosis and two years before we met through our mutual friend Autumn, who shared Ronda's story with me. After Ronda heard my story and learned my name, Autumn quickly introduced us via email, knowing I needed the "real-time" empathetic support she could provide. Within days of that contact, Ronda began sending me the letters one at a time so I could read and savor those moments at a pace that would strengthen my spirit. Each letter acknowledged a different emotion I was feeling, or had already felt, on my journey and provided an accompanying message of comfort. The correspondence encouraged me and gave me a renewed perspective on life despite my ongoing health challenges. It became increasingly clear to the three of us that this book of "Dear Susan" letters should be published to benefit others like me facing a life-changing illness, as well as their caregiving families and friends.

On several separate occasions, Ronda survived devastating health concerns that required prolonged time in bed. She persevered through the distressing experience of being a primary caregiver who was also the one in need. She is intimately familiar with the grief and anguish associated with a condition that may never be healed and a life that may never look quite the same.

But, more importantly, Ronda knows her God. She understands His compassion for us never fails and recognizes His internal leading in her spirit. Ronda knows that God's help is present for every trial we endure, and she relates His love in such a way that those who listen to her message can receive His peace even when mired in the fog of terrible circumstances.

Maybe you are not coping with a life-changing illness, but your world has come crashing down around you for another reason. Whether it is a bitter divorce, the loss of a child, financial ruin, or any number of other crises you might face, suffering is a universal phenomenon. At some point in each of our lives, a problem will arise that causes all other adversities to pale in comparison. In that moment, each of us needs someone who comprehends the raw emotions we encounter and can supply God-given wisdom born out of hard-won experience.

This book will guide you or a supportive friend or family member through the struggle, becoming a bridge to comfort, peace, and hope in the midst of pain. There are many self-help books and devotional journals in the marketplace, but none that brings comfort like this thoughtful collection gathered in the school of personal suffering. In these pages, you will find help, healing, and grace for the hardships you face today.

Susan Neibel, RN

A NOTE TO CAREGIVERS, FAMILY, AND FRIENDS

Dear Caregiver, Family Member, or Friend,

This book provides tangible pathways for processing feelings and fears accompanying the many struggles that come while living with a life-altering sickness. Perhaps you know or may be caring for such a loved one and are gifting this book to them. In these pages, you will find a poignant guide putting "words to feelings" often encountered "day-to-day" while grappling with the intensity of a debilitating illness.

I was blessed to be a caregiver to my dear friend, Susan. We both found these letters beneficial, as we navigated not only her feelings and struggles but my own as well. This book allowed us to take that journey together, entering a sacred place of communication, which alleviated the "what-ifs" and the daunting pressure of the unknown. The letters opened conversations addressing what might otherwise have been awkward "elephant in the room" topics and facilitated dialogue around our anxieties and heartfelt burdens.

As a caregiver, it is difficult to watch a loved one suffer, ultimately knowing you are unable to fix what's afflicting their physical body. However, having a template of specific subjects to discuss together is most comforting, as you individually face the intensity of the emotions that accompany the daily trials of illness, which often escalates during their care.

What a beautiful pathway you will walk, as you navigate this difficult journey together. Take the risk and be fully present, as you may be the only one who can listen to their heart, and care for your own in the process. Don't miss the glory shared in a most unlikely place.

Autumn Ross

A NOTE TO THE READER

This book would not be complete without the story of how I began writing letters to Susan. I see it as nothing less than a miracle that blessed me with a precious friendship and forever changed my life.

On a warm spring afternoon in 2017, I was standing in a bookstore when I overheard a customer ask the store clerk for a recommendation. The woman wanted a book for a friend who would undergo a bone marrow transplant within days. Tears filled her eyes as she explained that her dear friend would be in isolation for thirty days. She whispered, "I won't be able to see her, and I want to send a book she can take with her that will bring comfort and hope."

The love in the woman's eyes turned to desperation when the clerk replied, "I honestly can't think of anything."

My mind raced for ideas, and although I am a counselor and have endured my own long road with illness, neither was I aware of any helpful materials or resources that would provide what this lady wanted for her friend.

As I drove home, I felt angry. *"There should be a book! Why isn't there a book?"* I thought.

Almost immediately, God spoke to my heart, "Why don't you write one?"

I laughed and said out loud, "Me? I am not a writer!" Deep in my heart, however, I knew my personal journey with crushing illness had given me many experiences and words of comfort to share.

As the days turned into weeks and then months, the question, "Why don't you write one?" lingered in my heart. I couldn't get away from it. Finally, in the summer of 2018, I sat down to begin writing an initial draft. As if writing to a dear friend, my words took the form of a series of letters. I asked God for a name of someone to whom I could write, and the name "Susan" kept coming to mind. Soon, I began penning letters to Susan.

Each note of personal correspondence focused on an emotion my imaginary Susan might be feeling, such as fear, isolation, or guilt, and then guided her in processing that emotion. I wrote more than thirty letters to "Susan," and they quietly stayed in my journal for two years. Then, in June 2020, my friend Autumn told me about one of her dear friends who had been diagnosed with a terminal illness the summer I began writing the letters. She explained her friend had recently been sent home on hospice.

When I learned that the woman's name was Susan, I almost dropped the phone! I told Autumn about the letters in my journal and offered to send them to her. She told Susan about them and made a quick introduction.

One by one, I emailed the letters to both Susan and Autumn. As Susan read each letter, she responded. Together, Autumn and I learned so much about this extraordinary woman and her emotional experience in the face of pain, loss, and the unknown. In some small way, I was able to affirm her emotional journey, and she in turn affirmed the content and heart of the letters that had sat waiting in my journal for two long years. It became a beautiful exchange of two women acknowledging each other's journey through pain and suffering.

Dear friend, I have a question for you. Are you a Susan? If you are facing the pain and loss of a life-changing illness, and you fear the unknown, I wrote these letters for you. With each letter, I have included a journal page where you, too, can write and respond to each letter. It can be your private space, or you may share your thoughts and feelings with a caregiver, family member, or friend – just as Susan did.

Whatever you choose, please use that sacred journaling space to reflect, process, cry, laugh, grieve, or dream. Whatever you need to do. It is your letter. It is your story, your pain, your personal road to healing. May these letters provide comfort, hope, and peace as they remind you that you are not alone. I wrote them with this goal—and with you—in mind.

Thank you for joining me in this space. Let's journey together.

LET ME INTRODUCE MYSELF

Dear Susan,

You don't know me, but I have spent the past twenty years learning about you through my own healing journey. My learning comes out of the anguish, unexpected joys, countless tears, and times of deep soul searching that can only be done in the trenches and through the crucible of personal pain. I want you to know, I see you. I hear you. I feel with you.

I couldn't have written these letters 20 years ago, because I had not faced an illness that turns one's world upside down. While no two roads are exactly alike, I would like to walk yours with you. I am here to acknowledge and honor your journey, as well as offer love and support as you walk this difficult path.

As you read, dear friend, I hope these letters will give you a space to process your emotions and pain, offering you a place of hope and insight as real and honest as the emotions you are feeling. I am not here to give you pat answers, reasons, or formulas. In my experience, they are not helpful and more often, hurtful. My heart's desire is to simply sit with you in the middle of your suffering, acknowledge your pain, and remind you that you are not alone.

May you read these letters knowing I have you in mind. They come from a place of love for you with the humble knowledge that there may be things that don't apply to your life or circumstances. Please take what resonates with you and leave the rest. Ultimately, my prayer is that you will experience emotional honesty and comfort that awakens hope and gives you the freedom and strength to live your story fully alive.

I know you don't know me, yet, but I want you to know that I love you and that I care. It would be an honor and privilege to be with you through your suffering. May we walk together?

With a heart of love for you,

Ronda

THE STORY OF MY HEART

Dear Susan,

As we begin this journey together, I want to share with you a bit of my personal experience with a life-changing illness. Recognizing we all have our unique medical stories, instead of giving you the details of my diagnosis and treatments, I want to give you a window into the pain and loss I have experienced. As you read, please know this. Sharing experiences is not about comparing stories or scars: pain is pain; loss is loss; grief is grief. No one wants the trophy. And there is no reason to minimize our pain because someone else has "more." How is "more" even measured? Another's pain doesn't legitimize or negate our suffering. This has been a hard lesson but freeing on many levels.

That said, there are many experiences I have not encountered. But upon reflection, these are some of the things my heart has deeply felt. This is what my soul knows . . .

I know what it is like to have your world turned upside down . . . to desperately want what was . . . to have your health back. I know what it is like to want the norm . . . that which has been lost. I know what it is like to watch others easily go on with their lives and have the strength to do things they seem to take for granted or even dread, and yet, you would love to walk in their shoes and experience their health for just one day. I know what it is like to feel as though no one really understands not having the option to go to the grocery store, do laundry, or even sit up for long periods of time. Feeling as though no one understands is a lonely place. I know what it is like to feel you are a burden . . . to not be able to contribute to your family, to not be able to volunteer at your child's school, or to prepare a meal for a sick friend because <u>you</u> are the sick friend. I know what it feels like to look in the mirror and not recognize the reflection looking back at you because your body has become so emaciated, pale, and frail despite how hard you fight the disease. I know what it is like to endure pain day after day and have no hope it will ever stop or improve. I know what it is like to feel as though you are a failure as a wife because you are watching your husband desperately try to hold it all together when there is nothing you can do to ease his burden. I know what it is like to feel as though you are a failure as a parent . . . to not be able to run with your children at the playground or shop for them as they outgrow their clothes. I know what it feels like to wonder whether you matter anymore. I know what it is like to feel half dead and only partially alive. I know what it is like to wonder if you will survive and see your children grow into adulthood . . . wondering if you will be there to teach and guide them is excruciating. I know what it is like to feel completely out of control . . . unable to predict your ability to do anything because you never know what your body will allow. I know what it is like to lose the respect of others, especially doctors, who don't understand. I know what it is like for medical professionals not to see the vibrant real you who wants to be well again. They are unable to see how far you have fallen. They seem to only see a weak, frail, helpless, sick person who they don't really know how to help. I know what it is like to feel vulnerable and to be personally stripped down until there is nothing left to strip. I know what it is like to feel desperate . . . to be willing to do anything or go anywhere to find the answers that will lead to healing. I know what it feels like to give up . . . to see no end to the pain . . . no end to the desperation. I know what it is like to feel defeated and exhausted because the answers are not giving any relief. I know what it is like to feel angry . . . so angry that life isn't working out the way I had planned.

I know what it feels like to wonder, *"Why?"* I know . . .

Dear friend, what does your heart know? Use the next page to write what your soul knows.

Love,

Ronda

JOURNAL

What my soul knows ...

....
....
....
....
....
....
....
....
....
....
....
....
....
....
....
....
....
....
....
....
....
....
....

YOU ARE NOT A BURDEN

Dear Susan,

When you are dealing with illness, you can feel like a burden. Oh yes, a big, complicated, needy burden! You don't want to be an imposition to your family and friends, but the fact is, right now, you have needs – both big and small – that can feel like a heavy weight.

It is hard to have needs and be dependent on others – even when you know they care. You feel vulnerable as you find yourself unable to control or predict even the simplest of things in your day. Yes, it is unsettling to be the one asking for help. At times, it is even hard to know what would bring relief or how to give voice to it, so you don't speak up or reach out for what you need. Even when you do ask, it can be even harder to receive. Every act of kindness and love is humbling, and in a twisted way, frustrating – especially when you have always been the caregiver.

Dear friend, I get it. I remember times of deep sadness and frustration when I had to ask for help. My heart resisted being dependent on someone else for what I "should" be able to do. The shoulds of my mind were many, and they perpetuated a sense of shame and embarrassment for even having needs.

However, I came to realize that needs are not shameful. They are a beautiful and necessary part of the human experience representing avenues of connection, love, and healing. Accepting them as such is key to seeing ourselves as worthy of having needs and graciously receiving.

Friend, you are worthy of healing and love. Your view of yourself in the equation is so important. Thank your caregivers as the hands and feet of Love. Allow them to care for you. Let them wrap you in compassion and kindness. Don't hate or despise your need for them.

You see, the truth is we are interdependent, and we are walking each other home. Yes, we need each other. We are all a part of one body. The Bible encourages us to bear each other's burdens and in so doing, fulfill the law of Christ. What is Christ's law? Love. When we allow others to serve us, we partake in a beautiful transaction of love. You are not a burden. You are loved. You are human, and humans have messy, beautiful needs.

Allow love to be a balm that heals your body and soul.

With a heart of love for you!

Ronda

....

"Bear one another's burdens, and thereby fulfill the law of Christ," **Gal 6:2 (NASB)**.

JOURNAL

How do you view your needs?

....
....
....
....
....
....
....
....
....
....
....
....
....
....
....
....
....
....
....
....

DO YOU FEEL INVISIBLE?

Dear Susan,

Today, you feel invisible. People walk by you, but they don't see. No one knows. They don't realize the deep pain you carry or understand your loss. How could they? You don't have the strength or words to tell them. You feel alone, unseen. The illness has caused the life you once knew to disappear and somehow, it feels as though you disappeared with it. Many days, you feel known by your diagnosis as if it is a banner you wear, or you may struggle with an illness that is not apparent to those you meet. Whatever your case, the dignity of being seen, known, and understood has been silently ripped away, and yes, you feel invisible.

You no longer walk through this world in the role you once played. You remember being the life of the party, or the one whom family and friends counted on to be the organizer, caregiver, volunteer, or adventurer. It is as if you have been a victim of identity theft. You don't recognize the reflection in the mirror, and you aren't sure who you are anymore.

You experience pain in the confines of your heart, hospital bed, or home. Yes, it is felt deeply in the privacy of your soul, and you've become unable or afraid to express the sorrow harbored there. There is so much pain that is unseen and unknown.

I will never forget one particularly dark, early morning when I arrived early for a medical appointment. As I sat in my car in the parking lot, I watched hospital employees arrive to begin their shifts. I remembered the days I too walked into a hospital to begin my workday, and I cried. I cried tears of sadness and loss, and I felt invisible. It was as if the life I once knew had been erased, and with it, I was somehow erased as well.

Oh, my dear friend, if you resonate with my words, know I see you. As I write this, I cry with you. And in this moment, my heart firmly knows, if I can see you, there is also One who sees you perfectly.

Yes, He sees the real you, not just the role you once played. You have not disappeared. The Creator knows your name and every hair on your head (or no longer on your head). You are not invisible. My dear friend, may you know this truth today. You are seen and loved. So, SO loved.

With a heart of love that sees you!

Ronda

....

"Are not five sparrows sold for two cents? Yet not one of them is forgotten before God. Indeed, the very hairs of your head are all numbered. Do not fear; you are more valuable than many sparrows," **Luke 12:6-7 (NASB).**

....

"O Lord, You have searched me and known me. You know when I sit down and when I rise up; You understand my thought from afar. You scrutinize my path and my lying down, and are intimately acquainted with all my ways," **Ps 139:1-3 (NASB).**

JOURNAL

What do you want people to know and
understand about you?

....

....

....

....

....

....

....

....

....

....

....

....

....

....

....

....

....

....

....

IT'S OK TO GRIEVE

Dear Susan,

Do you feel a deep sense of sadness and loss? If so, you may be experiencing grief. You can't shake it off or ignore it. You can't escape it. Everywhere you look, you see devastation, loss of what was and uncertainty of what will be. Life will never be the same. You can't undo it, but how you wish you could. What you see before you is nothing like you have ever known. You want your life back. Dear friend, I hear you and feel your deep sense of loss. It is so painful.

A few years ago, I went to the beach with a few close girlfriends. It was gorgeous, tranquil, and ideal in every way! I wanted to share this paradise with my family. When I got home, I convinced my husband to go, and we immediately booked our flights with great anticipation!

A few weeks before we were to leave, a hurricane hit the coast. We waited anxiously to hear how our vacation destination fared. Fortunately, even though it sustained damage, my dream beach would reopen. We arrived knowing we would find damage, but I was not prepared for what I saw.

"Mom, is this what you brought us here to see?" my daughter asked as we looked down the debris-littered shoreline of my paradise beach. Much of the beach was gone and the stench was awful! My expectations of utopia had evaporated. All my glorious memories of what "was" were not sufficient to overcome the loss of the reality before us.

The beauty I wanted to share with my family was gone, and I knew the truth. The beach I had experienced would never be exactly the same. I sat and cried. As I wept, I couldn't understand the intensity of my tears until I realized this was a tangible picture of the loss I had felt with my physical health.

I had always been extremely healthy. My health had been a beautiful beach I wanted to share. However, when my kids were very young, a hurricane hit, leaving me with devastation. I tried my best to return my "beach" to its former glory. I wanted my kids to know the healthy me, but I have come to realize the only version they need from me is the one that presently exists.

Yes, my beach has changed. But as I have grieved the loss of what was, it has given me room to accept the beauty of the new before me. I walk on a new beach, and I have found treasures washed ashore that I did not see before.

With a heart of love for you!

Ronda

....

"I will give you the treasures of darkness, And hidden wealth of secret places, In order that you may know that it is I, The Lord, the God of Israel, who calls you by your name," **Isa 45:3 (NASB).**

JOURNAL

How has your beach changed, and what are you grieving?

....
....
....
....
....
....
....
....
....
....
....
....
....
....
....
....
....
....
....

HERE'S A RED RIBBON
OF HOPE

Dear Susan,

Today, you may feel like you have been turned inside out. Your life is upside down, and you are afraid it will never be the same. It is dark, and you feel yourself slipping into despair. As you search and grasp for normal, you have gnawing doubts, and you wonder if there is hope. It may feel as though you are holding the end of a rope, and your hands are slipping. It is as if you are suspended between life and death, and you aren't sure how long you can hang on to hope.

Oh, sweet friend, I too have faced dark days of wondering. It felt as though disease had stripped away my life, and I didn't know how to continue – just existing. I wanted to hang on, but so many times, my hands slipped. I knew if I let go, I would fall into utter hopelessness and would not survive. Letting go meant giving up, and in complete despair, I would not thrive – either emotionally or physically. But how long could I endure all this pain with no answers and with no end in sight? How long?

During that dark time, a friend of a friend sent me a beautiful card with a simple red ribbon accompanying the biblical story of Rahab from the Old Testament. Her story reminded me of how she put the red cord outside her window as the spies had instructed. It was a symbol that even in the middle of destruction, she would be held, safe and secure in God's care.

Though the city walls fell all around her, Rahab was safe. How scary it must have been when she heard the support under her feet crack, watching all she had once known crumble and disappear. In the middle of the devastation, I wonder if she experienced moments of hopelessness and fear? She may have wondered if she would survive. But when the dust settled, the red cord remained in her window as a symbol of hope. Despite the loss and devastation, God held her in his care.

I read Rahab's story with tears running down my face because I knew God also held me. I put my red ribbon of hope on my kitchen windowsill as a daily reminder that even though I didn't know how, when, or if I would find the healing I so desired, my Creator held me safe in the midst of all that seemed completely hopeless. As I looked at my red ribbon of hope, I began to realize it wasn't about me desperately holding onto hope, it was knowing that in the middle of loss and devastation, I am the one being held. Hope holds me.

Oh, dear friend, in the middle of your circumstances, you too are held. Always know, <u>you</u> are forever in His care, and you are so loved.

With a heart of love for you!

Ronda

....

"My soul clings to You; Your right hand upholds me," **Ps 63:8 (NASB).**

JOURNAL

What reminds you that you are held
by Hope?

....
....
....
....
....
....
....
....
....
....
....
....
....
....
....
....
....
....

THE TRUTH ABOUT FAILURE

Dear Susan,

Today, you may feel like you have let everyone down. Oh, friend, this is so hard. You are looking at all the boxes left unchecked, and you see the ideal in your mind of how it "should" be. You want the best for those you love, and you feel as though you have failed them or left them disappointed. What a painful place.

The rules of the game have changed. You are no longer the person your little ones call when they need help. You lie in bed listening to the hustle and bustle, and yet, cannot participate. To hear the people you love most struggle to keep it together and not be able to do it for them hurts. It is excruciating, and it feels like a deep, deep failure.

You don't like the new rules. You want to cry out and object, but for now, you can only sit with the disappointment and loss. This is not how you imagined life or your role as a spouse, parent, daughter, aunt, or friend to be. You blame yourself, your body, your choices, your doctors, even God. There must be someone to hold responsible. Your world is not right, and today, you accuse yourself. Yes, your finger is pointing inward.

Dear friend, when we experience pain, it can feel as though someone has to be blamed. We seek to understand why the suffering is happening, somehow fix it, and not let it happen again. Our minds try to make sense of it all by asking, "How did this happen?" "Who is at fault?"

However, remember, blame brings shame and despair. Truth brings freedom and life. While not what you imagined, knowing the complete truth about today can change your perspective and choices, allowing you to live in the beauty of it as well as in the loss.

The truth is you are still here. You can smile. You can love. You can pray. You can be YOU. You may not be able to find the tennis shoes or the lost socks, feed the dog, or drive to the store for milk, but you can still love. You still care. Otherwise, you wouldn't feel this deep loss or try to fix it.

The truth is you are a gift. The packaging may look a bit different, but as long as you have breath, your life has significance. You have so much to offer. Your family needs your love, your warmth, and your care. They need <u>you</u>. They don't need your cooking, organizational skills, or other capabilities as much as they need who you are as a unique individual. You are more than what you do. You, my dear friend, are a human being, not a human doing, and you continue to create beauty in this world with your very presence. Influence, impact, and precious memories are not measured by strength and action, they are created by your love.

You have not failed. Don't let blame rob you of the gifts you bring. Give yourself compassion and empathy. You haven't let them down. Rather, you lift them up with your presence and love.

You, my precious friend, are enough.

With a heart of deep love for you!

Ronda

....

"Love never fails...," **I Cor 13:8a (NIV).**

JOURNAL

How do you bring love and influence
into the lives of those you touch?

....

....

....

....

....

....

....

....

....

....

....

....

....

....

....

....

....

....

....

TIRED OF THE FEAR

Dear Susan,

Today, you may feel afraid; you fear the unknown and the "what-ifs". You have never walked this path before, and all you see is disappointment and loss.

How did you get here? How can this be your story? What will tomorrow bring? With so much pain and devastation, it is difficult to think tomorrow will be any different. How can you hope to see goodness when you trusted before and have been left with such a deep sense of devastation and loss?

The loss you feel is oh, so deep. You can't see the bottom. If you allowed yourself to feel the depths of it, you fear this pit would consume you in utter darkness.

You try to push it all away but are haunted by the voices in your head and the pain in your heart. You long to know peace and rest, but the reality of disappointment and loss screams to be heard. You feel the injustice of it all. The things for which you had hoped, you do not see. In the silence, you remember the moment when hope was lost. Now, you walk a path you have never taken before, and instead of hope being your companion, you face fear – seemingly abandoned and alone.

Oh, friend, I am sorry you find yourself in this dark place. You don't know what is ahead, and you aren't sure where Love is right now. Please know this . . . Love is never absent. Love holds you in the darkness, the loss, the questions, the disappointment. Love is able. Love enters in with you and shines a light into the darkness as only Love can do because God is Love.

Don't be afraid to feel deep emotions and ask painful questions. When you avoid difficult feelings, you shut them all away – even pleasant ones. You can't outrun fear, disappointment, or loss.

When you face the darkness, you won't do it alone. Love will be there, and you will see it perfected in the very place you feared to go. Love goes with you to face the fear. Yes, Love touches our fear and brings healing truth, courage, and a place of shelter from the storm. Perfect Love does cast out fear. In the middle of the unknown, Love will be the companion to light your path.

With a heart of love for you!

"There is no fear in love; but perfect love casts out fear . . ." **I John 4:18a (NASB).**

"Trust in him at all times, you people; pour out your hearts to Him, for God is our refuge," **Ps 62:8 (NIV).**

JOURNAL

What emotions and questions are you afraid to face?

....

....

....

....

....

....

....

....

....

....

....

....

....

....

....

....

....

....

....

MOVING FROM FROZEN TO FORWARD

Dear Susan,

Today, you feel frozen. There are so many voices telling you what to do and many of them contradict or even oppose each other. To whom do you listen? Which direction should you go? What steps do you take? Which path will lead to healing? Which voice has a bias or agenda? Do they really know and understand? You don't know and can't discern, and you feel frozen.

I always believed my doctor or specialist had the answers, and as a medical professional, I trusted my colleagues for the solution. Yes, I firmly believed that the medical experts around me would be able to provide a diagnosis, relief, or remedy, as needed.

When I became ill, that belief failed me. No one had an answer or even a guess that brought healing, or at the very least, a measure of relief. They wanted to help, but they didn't know. Their experience had not prepared them for the complexity of what my body faced. I wanted someone to stand up and say, "I have the answer. Just do this!" or, "Here are 10 things. Do them, and you will get better." Over time, I realized I was on my own. I felt lost, confused, angry, and frozen.

I discovered there were solutions, but one doctor alone couldn't "fix" my problem. I began to look to the Great Physician, the One who created every cell and sustains every breath I breathe. I depended on Him to guide me through this confusing maze. I asked for direction, and in the quiet of my moments, His still small voice gave me direction. Not an audible voice, but an impression in my spirit or an idea to pursue. Someone would suggest a doctor, hand me a book, or a website that would resonate with me. I stayed open to learning and listening.

Though big steps were sometimes necessary, listening and taking consistent small steps one at a time moved me from frozen to forward and brought healing. Have I done it perfectly? Absolutely not! Have I tried things and not seen the benefit I hoped? Yes, but it doesn't mean they didn't prove to be useful pieces of the puzzle.

If you are looking to flawlessly execute the perfect path, you won't find it and will remain frozen. However, if you start with stillness and listen to the One who created you and knows your name, you can begin walking. Even if you are not sure where the path will end or if you can complete the journey, just take the next step. Yes, in all of its imperfection, lean into this moment – just do today. It is enough.

With a heart of love for you!

Ronda

....

"I will instruct you and teach you in the way which you should go; I will counsel you with My eye upon you," **Ps 32:8 (NASB).**

JOURNAL

What is your next step that will take you from frozen to forward, healing motion?

....
....
....
....
....
....
....
....
....
....
....
....
....
....
....
....
....
....
....
....

THIS IS NOT PUNISHMENT

Dear Susan,

You are suffering and there is something you need to know – you are not being punished. What a debilitating and agonizing thought and a horrible lie. To think your condition is punitive is unthinkable. My heart longs for you to hear me. I know the recordings that play in your mind. *Did I do something wrong? Just tell me, and I will apologize.*

Does God really play hide and seek and leave us wondering what in the world we did to deserve this? Or maybe, you think you know what you did, and an accusing and condemning voice in your head torments you, reminding you of every infraction, indiscretion, or poor choice.

Oh, friend, if you hear nothing else, hear this. Your pain or illness is not punishment! God has no need or desire to punish you. Would you allow someone you love to be tortured because of something they did? Is that how you would reconcile a wrong?

There is good news. Wrongs are always reconciled through forgiveness and love. You are no exception. You, my dear friend, are both forgiven and so loved. Love always comes for you. Those words may be bouncing off you right now, and you may wish you could feel and truly experience them. Whether you believe them or not, they are true. Say it out loud. Write it in your journal. Allow these thoughts to be your mantra until your heart believes and experiences its truth, "I am forgiven and uncon-ditionally loved."

Forgiveness has already happened. Whatever the offense, as far as the east is from the west, it is removed from you. While acknowledging wrong is the first step toward truth and healing, you don't have to hold on to it. It is not a life sentence to be paid with regret, shame, and condemnation. You are free. Now, forgive yourself; let the weight of it go.

Yes, some choices bring natural consequences that are painful. Brokenness begets pain. As part of the human race, you will be touched by brokenness and heartache. This is a harsh reality of the human condition. However, it should never be interpreted as punishment or restitution.

There is no payment required. It is called grace. Welcome to grace and love. Taste this healing balm. They wait for you with open arms and the embrace of a Father who is asking you to come and sit at His table, to drink, eat, and rest in His love.

You are not being punished. He delights in you. He loves you. Stop punishing yourself. It won't make you feel better, and it will never be enough. Let yourself heal in the light and truth of forgiveness, love, and grace. Let go of the chains of punishment and regret, and walk free.

With a heart of love for you!

Ronda

....

"As far as the east is from the west, So far has He removed our transgressions from us," **Ps 103:12 (NASB).**

JOURNAL

What ideas about punishment or con-
demnation hold you hostage? Take time
to reflect on how truth, love, and grace
can free you.

....
....
....
....
....
....
....
....
....
....
....
....
....
....
....
....
....
....

LET ME TELL YOU
MY GREATEST FEAR

Dear Susan,

There may be days when you experience anxiety and fear. Their weight can drain your energy, steal your joy, and keep you confused and overwhelmed. You could write a list of fears that rob you of peace. But there is one that is especially hard to face. You can hardly bear or speak of it, but it weighs heavy on you. My friend, can you name it? What is your greatest fear?

Mine was not being here to raise my children, for my children not to know me, and to feel abandoned.

Yep! Hands down, leaving my children motherless has been my greatest fear. It taunted me. It raised its loud voice at every turn with all the "what-ifs". The illness reminded me I am mortal; there are no guarantees. I couldn't escape the fear. It had a grip on me and tried to rob me of the beauty and joy that I did have in motherhood.

I began to view fear as a failure and a foe, but it is neither. Like every other emotion, it is a messenger giving us information. Fear alerts us to danger, so we can fight, freeze, or run to safety. Acknowledging and understanding its presence and message is so important. Strength and courage are not synonymous with avoiding or stuffing emotions. That is why God acknowledges fear, speaks words of peace, and reminds us we are not alone. He is with us – always.

To feel afraid is part of the human experience. It is when we carry the threat day after day that we are robbed of peace. We begin to live as though there is no place to run or hide, no solace for the weary, or shelter from the storm. Instead of a temporary alert, fear can become a constant voice, and our body stays in a perpetual state of hypervigilance, keeping us narrowly focused on all the possible threats.

Fear is a funny thing. It shouts to convince you that its threats are reality – a done deal. It overrides the truth of the present.

Your body responds to this fear as if it is your absolute reality. It creates a fight-or-flight response and brings stress. At a time when you most need rest, comfort, and peace, it hijacks your body and makes you a slave to its bidding.

We often fear the things we believe would be beyond our ability to tolerate or cope. For us, it is the unthinkable. We try to hide or avoid it. Yet, it consumes our thoughts, and we find ourselves staring at the very thing we long to forget.

Our greatest fear may also be the thing we consider a threat to what we hold most dear. These precious gifts are to be enjoyed and protected. But when we grasp them with the grip of fear or attempt to ensure what we cannot control, our love turns to fear, panic, and torment.

Dear friend, you won't ever be able to outrun the thing you fear most. It is the monster of the future. You are a citizen of this moment. Your mind can wander into the "what-ifs" of the future, but your body can only be in this present moment where

Love meets and holds you. When you abide in the certainty of this Love, and you release what you hold dear knowing it also abides in Love, you will find a place of rest.

Instead of fighting the dreaded unknowns of the future, let your mind join your body in the now. Be fully present. You don't have to live tormented by the thing you most fear. Fear lives in the distant future. You reside in the here and now where nothing can separate you from Love. Nothing. In this moment, Love greets you and holds you. And sweet friend, in the next now, Love will be there too.

Fear of the future will rob you blind and take everything you hold dear. Acknowledge and process the pain it reflects, but don't let it fester and grow. Don't let it dictate your thoughts. Love rules the now.

With a heart of love for you!

Ronda

....

"Do not fear, for I am with you; Do not anxiously look about you, for I am your God. I will strengthen you, surely I will help you, Surely I will uphold you with my righteous right hand," **Isa 41:10 (NASB).**

JOURNAL

When you think of your greatest fear,
what helps you stay present to this
moment where Love holds you?

....

....

....

....

....

....

....

....

....

....

....

....

....

....

....

....

....

....

AWAKEN TO HOPE

Dear Susan,

Where are you with hope today? Hope can be fragile - here one moment and shattered the next. Yet, it holds the power of life and death. Hope represents the longings of our heart, points to our deepest desires, and gives us the ability to keep going, keep walking, and rise above the impossible to live another day. The hope we felt yesterday shows us how to hope again.

When we don't secure the things for which we hope, we often feel hopeless. I know I have, and it was devastating. Without hope, we are lost and undone. We lose vision and don't know which way to turn. Hopeless, we often turn downward into despair. With no way out and no light at the end of the tunnel, we give up. We want the nightmare to end.

Oh, dear friend, I hear you. You have suffered so much. You are exhausted in every way possible, and to continue hoping requires energy you just cannot muster. You can't do it anymore. I have good news. You don't have to. You heard me right. Hope isn't something you lose. It is already and always there, and when you awaken to hope, you will recognize its evidence everywhere.

Hope is ...

- The very breath you breathe;

- The love that surrounds you every moment of the day;
- The voice inside that whispers, *"You are His"*;
- The beauty in each moment you live;
- The bright light and love you witness in those you love;
- The promise that there is purpose in the life you live today;
- A beating heart giving witness to the fact that you are fully alive;
- The desire to give and receive love;
- The knowing that you are never alone;
- The assurance that there is still goodness, yours for the taking;
- The knowing your future is secure and safe;
- The comfort you are His beloved and never out of His care;
- The recognition you can choose how to live the life you possess;
- The anticipation there are new miracles and mercies every morning.

Do you see, dear friend? Hope isn't something you must desperately try to secure. Hope secures you. Hope isn't about what you lose or keep. It is having eyes to see the reality of what you already possess and cannot be taken away.

Yes, hope ungirds us, and a heart awakened to hope accepts the urge to fly and simply spreads its wings.

With a heart of love for you!

Ronda

....

"Hope deferred makes the heart sick, but desire fulfilled is a tree of life," **Prov 13:12 (NASB).**

....

"And now, Lord, for what do I wait? My hope is in You," **Ps 39:7 (NASB).**

JOURNAL

Where do you see the evidence of hope around you?

....
....
....
....
....
....
....
....
....
....
....
....
....
....
....
....
....
....
....
....

THE MIND-BODY
CONNECTION

Dear Susan,

Today, you are in pain. SO. MUCH. PAIN. It is hard to tell where the relentless physical torment stops, and the emotional agony begins. You are hurting, and it goes so deep and wide. You're not even sure of the source or which is worse, the emotional anguish or the physical misery.

I hear you. You are right: it can be both. Yes, our bodies influence our emotions, and our emotions affect our bodies. You are living it. You feel the internal anguish as you experience the physical misery of the day-to-day. At times, it is so intense, it may be hard to distinguish between the two. They really do walk hand-in-hand and operate in conjunction with one another.

My dear friend, as I have walked my healing road, I have also experienced the reciprocal relationship between my mind and body. I experienced many symptoms that brought physical pain, and my primary focus was to alleviate my physical suffering. However, I noticed that as I began to process my emotional suffering, it took a heavy burden off my body, freeing energy and resources for healing. It allowed me to look at the "whole" me as I pursued wholeness.

My friend, as you seek care for your physical needs, look at your emotional needs as well. They matter and influence your healing. When you process painful emotions, you will give your body a gift of support and love. This does not imply emotions are shameful. Your feelings are neither good nor bad, wrong nor right, and they don't always reflect the full truth. They are important and essential information about how you are perceiving and experiencing your circumstances. Your emotions are a beautiful expression and reflection of your inner world. They are worthy of having a voice. Let them speak. Where do you feel your emotions in your body? Do you notice the sensations? What are your emotions trying to say? Listen, and let them be heard.

At times, it can be hard to understand and process it all alone. You may need someone to come alongside and help you sort through the emotions you are experiencing, which is perfectly natural. I strongly encourage you to seek out a professional counselor or life coach who works with individuals facing a life-changing illness. They can help you understand the intricate relationship between your mind and body and give you the space and tools to address it.

As you seek healing, don't forget to look at the whole – all of you. Maybe, it holds a key to healing. God created you as a beautifully interconnected system. Your sacred and unique path to physical healing may also involve spiritual and emotional healing.

There is only one of you. Walk open to complete healing as uniquely as YOU.

With a heart of love for you!

Ronda

....

"A happy heart is good medicine, and a joyful mind causes healing, But a broken spirit dries up the bones," **Prov 17:22 (AMP).**

....

"The human spirit can endure in sickness, but a crushed spirit who can bear?" **Prov 18:14 (NIV).**

JOURNAL

How has your illness affected you phys-
ically, emotionally, and spiritually?

....

....

....

....

....

....

....

....

....

....

....

....

....

....

....

....

....

....

....

ISOLATED BUT NOT ALONE

Dear Susan,

Illness can be isolating. It is easy to become isolated from family and friends because you can't keep up or are no longer able to go where they may be. Whether living at home, a hospital, rehab center, psychiatric facility, or nursing home, you are no longer able to participate in the life you once knew.

Dear friend, I know what it is like to hear about the parties, events, field trips, vacations, road trips, ball games, girls' nights out, Bible studies, promotions, and the lives that continue to go on while you feel stuck in time. It is lonely.

The loneliness stems from a lack of proximity, but it goes even deeper. You have a sense of isolation because no one can feel your exact pain. It feels as though it is yours alone to bear. No one can crawl in your skin and experience the physical and mental anguish of it all. They may care deeply, but they can't know. It is like your own secret held inside that no one else can completely understand. You want so badly for them to comprehend it. You don't want to be alone in it, but you wouldn't wish this pain on anyone. You've determined not to be the person always complaining, and you want to protect them from it, so you find yourself minimizing or ignoring how you feel. You don't want it to leak out on them or hurt them too, so you bear it alone. Yes, you feel alone in the grip and complexity of your private pain and anguish. You long for a place of honesty, vulnerability, connection, and understanding, but it eludes you.

My dear friend, I have come to understand that when God says He is present in our pain, He isn't kidding. He has not turned away from you, nor does He stand as a stoic witness. As One who knows sorrow and is acquainted with grief, He is a God who experiences our pain. Yes, He is in pain with you. He is not removed from it. Rather, He enters our pain – always. He is Immanuel, "God with us." That's what Love does. Take a moment and breathe in this truth. You are not alone in your experiences and suffering. My dear friend, you are not alone.

With a heart of love for you!

Ronda

....

"He was despised and rejected by men, a man of sorrows and acquainted with grief . . ." **Isa 53:3a (ESV).**

....

"Behold, the virgin shall be with child and shall bear a son, and they shall call His name Immanuel," which *translated means, 'God with us,'"* **Matt 1:23 (NASB).**

JOURNAL

How has isolation impacted you?

....
....
....
....
....
....
....
....
....
....
....
....
....
....
....
....
....
....
....
....
....
....

LET'S DANCE

Dear Susan,

You feel your life has stopped. It's as if someone pushed the pause button, and your life has been suspended. You are in a holding pattern, waiting for things to get back to normal. You are waiting for the pain, treatment, and symptoms to stop. When all of this is over, you can get back to your real life and begin to thrive again.

I remember thinking, *Once I get past this, I will be able to move beyond merely existing to again start "fully living."* It was as if I was holding my breath until it was over. Inside, my heart felt half dead as if I wasn't completely alive. I just wanted my real life back.

Then, one day, I read a quote from Vivian Greene that stopped me in my tracks. It completely shifted my perspective, for which I am so grateful. I bought a sign with the quote on it, making it my daily mantra:

*Life isn't about waiting for the storm to pass...
It's about learning to dance in the rain.*

I repeated those words in my mind and asked myself, "Is it possible to dance in the middle of the storm? Is it possible to find joy in the midst of suffering? How would that change my life?" I came to understand dancing didn't mean ignoring difficult emotions and only acknowledging the pleasant. No, dancing is the audacity to embrace the messiness, and live it all; taste it all; feel it all – the joy, pain, loss, and beauty. Both joy and sorrow are part of my real life, and I don't want to deny myself the opportunity to live my full story. Yes, living every messy drop of it is what it means to dance in the rain.

I remember the day I made a conscious decision to not merely survive, but purposely live my full story. I realized I didn't have to think of my circumstances as a time to close my eyes and hold my breath. This was my real life, and although not what I would have chosen, I didn't want to miss it. These difficult days were still my days, and I had a choice as to how I would participate in them. I might have felt "half dead," but I had a beating heart. I was alive, and I could live as such.

Looking back, I can see how those days quickly turned into months, and months became precious years. If I had not learned to dance, I would have missed out on priceless moments with my husband, growing children, extended family, and friends. I didn't dance perfectly, but I stopped waiting to dance. And as I breathed, I experienced the beauty of living with my heart – fully alive.

Oh, dear friend, I know there is a huge storm, and the pain can cast a dark shadow coloring everything gray. But I encourage you to open your eyes and see the full spectrum in your life. The rain doesn't tell your full story. There are spectacular hues of red, yellow, blue, and green. Let yourself feel and experience the loss and the joy. It is all a part of the beauty of your life. Don't deny yourself your full story – look up and see the full rainbow of color.

With a heart of love for you!

Ronda

....

"The Lord will command His loving kindness in the daytime, and His song will be with me in the night," **Ps 42:8 (NASB).**

JOURNAL

In the middle of your circumstances, what would it look like to dance in the rain?

....
....
....
....
....
....
....
....
....
....
....
....
....
....
....
....
....
....
....

EMBRACING
UNCONDITIONAL LOVE

Dear Susan,

There is something important you need to know today. You are loved. Yes, you! Can you sit with that statement? Can you let yourself feel it, hold it, and embrace it? You, my friend, are unconditionally loved.

The unconditional part is key. You see, love can only be experienced as love when given and received unconditionally. Love given or received in any other way violates the very nature of love. Your past, your state of mind, your circumstances – none of that matters. You are loveable just as you are.

I know the word "loveable" may feel foreign right now. I have been there. I remember feeling as if the rug had been pulled out from under me, and everything loveable about me went with it. How I portrayed myself to the world was gone. My body was altered, my energy diminished, and my ability to do even simple things was gone. I felt stripped bare with nothing left to cover me. Little did I know that this was a place of just being and receiving love.

Dear friend, if you find yourself in a similar mind-set, believe it or not, that is a powerful space. With the means for performance, achievements, pretense, and expectation gone, you are in a place to taste, receive, and embrace this beautiful gift of uncon-ditional love.

You see, even if love has previously been offered unconditionally, we often don't receive it that way. When we have something to offer, we depend— often unknowingly—on those things to earn love.

I know it may feel vulnerable, but this is the very place where heaven and earth meet. In this space our hearts can say, "Yes", and every cell of our bodies can receive and feel the love that has always been there. Finally, we can see the unconditional love we missed while we were busy making ourselves loveable.

Hey Susan, heaven and earth have met, and God wants you to know how dearly He loves you, in this moment and always. Like a messenger in first grade, I pass along this love note to you. I hope you check the box that says, "Yes, I accept!" May today be the day you receive love as an unconditional gift. You are precious. You are valued. You are loved for just being you!

With a heart full of love for you!

Ronda

....

"Who shall ever separate us from the love of Christ? Will tribulation, or distress, or persecution, or famine, or nakedness, or danger, or sword? . . . For I am convinced-beyond any doubt-that neither death, nor life, nor angels, nor principalities, nor things present and threatening, nor things to come nor powers, or height,

nor depth, nor any other created thing, will be able to separate us from the unlimited love of God which is in Christ Jesus our Lord," **Rom 8:35, 37-39 (AMP).**

JOURNAL

Tell me about your response to the invitation of unconditional love.

....
....
....
....
....
....
....
....
....
....
....
....
....
....
....
....
....
....
....
....
....

SETBACKS ARE SO HARD

Dear Susan,

Today, you may be facing a setback. Setbacks are so very hard. After taking two steps forward, it's disheartening to take three steps back.

I find myself there today as well. It is agonizing, frustrating, and sad. After gaining a bit of my old functionality and health, today, I struggle with this old reality.

I had grown fond of my new capabilities but right now, my body requires rest, grace, and compassion. Not that I don't need those things every day, but today, I need a little more.

Dear friend, I am sorry you find yourself in that place as well, but please know that there are better days ahead. I know the events of today can feel permanent, unending, and may overshadow everything else in your life, but they do not reflect the full story of your life.

Regardless of your circumstance, don't forget to live in the setback. This day holds beauty. It is still good. And in the middle of the setback, don't forget to be present, breathe, and embrace life today. There is so much more.

With a heart of love for you!

Ronda

....

"I will open rivers on the bare heights, And springs in the midst of the valley; I will make the wilderness a pool of water, and the dry land fountains of water," **Isa 41:18 (NASB).**

....

"I would have despaired unless I had believed that I would see the goodness of the Lord in the land of the living," **Ps 62:2 (NASB).**

JOURNAL

How can you take care of yourself while facing this setback?

....
....
....
....
....
....
....
....
....
....
....
....
....
....
....
....
....
....
....
....
....
....

CAN YOU DO THIS MOMENT?

Dear Susan,

You have had enough. You just can't do it anymore. You have hit a wall and don't have the strength to get through this month, this week, or even this day. You are exhausted and feel the heaviness of despair.

Oh, dear friend, I am so sorry. There was a day when I too was at the end. I was only going through the motions of existing, and I was exhausted. Afraid and in debilitating pain, fog surrounded my brain. Weeks had turned into years, and I just couldn't do it anymore. The prospect of facing this life for the unknown future left me overwhelmed and in deep despair. I just couldn't continue to go on.

I will never forget a pivotal afternoon. I made the painful journey from my bed to the refrigerator in an attempt to give my body a bit of nutrition. I opened the door, and nothing made sense. As a dietitian, I always found a measure of assurance in the fact that I knew how to give my body nourishment. It was the one thing I could do for myself. But there I stood, with a refrigerator full of food, at a complete loss. Who was I? This is how I help others, and I couldn't even help myself. I had hit a wall!

I closed the refrigerator door in complete despair. The weight of my weak body leaned on the cold stainless-steel refrigerator for support, and I cried out with tears flowing down my face, "I can't do this anymore!" All I could hear were my own sobs.

In my despair, God unexpectedly placed a question in my heart, "Can you do this moment?"

The question caught me off guard, but as I pondered it, everything narrowed to that single second in time. I was able to be present in that very moment, and unexpectedly, I felt a sense of relief. Yes, the moment was painfully hard, but doable, even bearable.

I uttered with a whisper, "Yes, I can do this moment, but I don't know if I can do two seconds from now. And only if You hold me; only if I am not alone."

My heart heard an assurance, "I am holding you in this moment. And all your future moments, I will be holding them too."

I realized it wasn't the moment that was so unbearable. It was the weight of the unknown and trying to predict the future that was taking me under.

That day I learned to live in a way I had never known before – in the moment. I discovered that in the moment, there was always enough. It was fear of the future "what-ifs" that brought torture and despair. But when I allowed myself to experience and be present in the moment, I found relief and peace.

This new way of living also brought unexpected joy and rest. As a mom of young children, I knew my strength and steps were limited and each of them mattered if I were to care for my family. I began asking God how I should spend my moments. I couldn't discern what was most important or what lay ahead, but He knew, and I wanted Him to make my steps count.

Moment by moment, I asked God for the next step, and a thought or a quiet knowing would come. I'd get a nudge to sweep the floor or check my email, read a book, or simply rest.

The moment didn't usually look like what I would have ordered or planned, but as I let go of my plan and my expectations, I was able to receive, hold, and be present in the beauty of the moment. It brought joy and gratitude to really "see" my moments, and knowing God directed my steps, allowed me to rest. So, I lived my life - moment by moment.

May I leave you with this question, weary friend? Can you do this moment? I am not asking if you can do tomorrow, next week, or even two seconds from now. Breathe. Be here in this moment.

With a heart of love for you!

Ronda

....

"So do not worry about tomorrow; for tomorrow will care for itself. Each day has enough trouble of its own," **Matt 6:34 (NASB).**

JOURNAL

How does your heart hear the question,
"Can you do this moment?"

....
....
....
....
....
....
....
....
....
....
....
....
....
....
....
....
....
....
....

JOY, AN INSIDE JOB

Dear Susan,

Does your heart ever yearn for joy? The feeling of joy may seem like a distant memory, something that eludes you, or a frivolous extra. After all, you are just trying to get through this day and survive.

You may also think joy is for other people, and not for someone in your circumstance. It is for the strong and those who have their energy and health. At least for today, it doesn't sound like it is an option for you. If you achieve the level of health and vitality or dreams you desire, then, and only then, will joy again be a companion in your life. Oh, dear friend, I hear your heart.

A few years ago, I left wooden letters J-O-Y, wrapped in red velvet, over my kitchen sink all year long. I thought if I studied the Christmas decoration, osmosis would somehow allow joy to flood my heart.

You see, even before I fell ill, joy was a fleeting feeling that came and went, and after, it felt like a pipe dream. Me, joyous? I didn't think I had any reason to be joyous. All I saw before me was pain and loss. Sadness had moved in and laid claim to my heart. It wasn't always a horrible sadness. On most days, it was a dull sadness, but it made me feel dead inside. Vibrancy and the joy of living had crept away, and I wasn't sure they would ever return. So, I stared at the big, red velvet word over my sink pining for what seemed impossible.

Being ill can certainly change your perspective. My life had become very small, and there were many things I could no longer do. Finding joy in my career, exercise, an achievement, or the excitement of an adventurous trip was no longer an option for me. If I were to find joy, I knew it would somehow be discovered in the current circumstances of here and now.

On a daily basis, my little world consisted of my beautiful family. I had a wonderful husband, two amazing kids, and a comfortable home to call our own. Yes, in many ways, I had it all, but where was my joy? Was I defective?

I will never forget the evening when I unexpectedly encountered joy. I had achieved the rarity of being able to join my family for dinner. As I sat at the table, I was so thankful to simply be with them. Before being ill, I would have critiqued the food and judged my kids' table manners and dinner topics, but not on this day. I saw things very differently. I was simply taking in the faces I so loved, and it hit me like a bountiful, bubbling river flowing through my heart . . . joy!

I sat still basking in the feeling of joy, afraid the magic would disappear if I moved out of my chair. I had no expectations for that dinner, nor was I judging the moment. Instead, I felt a deep appreciation to be out of bed and eating with them. From this place of acceptance and gratitude, joy bubbled up inside of me. It wasn't forced; it simply and unexpectedly appeared as a beautiful gift to my heart.

The pain hadn't subsided, and I needed to rest, but joy gave me a deep, renewed inner strength, and I had eyes to see my life from a different vantage point.

I learned joy is not based on my circumstances or health. Instead, joy flows from a sense of awe and gratitude that is free of my own judgments. It is pure, authentic, not contrived, and brings incredible resilience and strength. Of course, there were (and are) still days of sadness, but I learned deep joy can appear like a refreshing drink of water in the desert of pain and sorrow.

I also learned joy is not based on other people's actions or perspectives. It comes from eyes willing to see and ears ready to hear. Joy cannot be taken away because it doesn't belong to or come from others. They may participate or be a catalyst, but joy comes from within.

Yes, dear friend, joy is an inside job, and it can appear in your world too. Don't judge. Embrace life with thankfulness and watch joy appear in the darkness.

With a heart of love for you!

Ronda

....

"Indeed, the Lord will comfort Zion; He will comfort all her waste places, And her wilderness He will make like Eden, and her desert like the garden of the Lord; Joy and gladness will be found in her, Thanksgiving and sound of a melody." **Isa 51:19 (NASB).**

JOURNAL

How can you invite joy into your life?

....
....
....
....
....
....
....
....
....
....
....
....
....
....
....
....
....
....
....

THE VALUE OF REST

Dear Susan,

Rest, my dear Susan. This concept can be so counter to our societal norm. Our culture glamorizes efficiency, productivity, hard work, and excess, while it downplays or outright ignores the dignity and necessity of rest. These are loud voices, but please, hear me. Rest is so very important. It is the state of repair and healing. It is a sacred space.

Even though you are experiencing illness, life goes on all around you. Its demands ring in your ears. With so much to do, you continue to push. You try to maintain the routines of life while your body struggles to keep up. You are so accustomed to responding to the crises of the day that you don't recognize your body's pleas for rest.

Rest can seem counterintuitive when you are in the fight for your life. You are pushing, fighting, and striving. The resulting flurry, panic, and frenzy give the illusion you are doing something. You are waging war against illness, and you will not let it win!

Dear friend, the passion to heal is fuel for hope, but don't confuse this passion with a state of crisis. Panic and striving leave your cells in a perpetual state of fight-or-flight. They create a place of crisis, a call to all-hands-on-deck. The cortisol rush that accompanies crisis is meant to be temporary. Staying in crisis mode will exhaust rather than repair your body. It is not a place of healing.

For most of my life, when I spoke of rest, it was in the context of a long nap or a good night's sleep. However, I learned if I wanted to experience complete rest, I couldn't ignore my emotional self. My body experienced true rest when I began to seek and value both emotional and physical rest.

Emotional rest is a place of safety, compassion, gratitude, and love. Can you sense the shift in your body when you feel these emotions? They align your mind and body allowing you to rest, restore, and heal. Yes, this is rest. It is a space free of bitterness and turmoil and full of forgiveness, acceptance, and peace. Rest may appear to be a passive state; however, it is purposeful, and it is oh, so powerful.

Yes, I said powerful. The need for rest does not mean you are weak. On the contrary, it gives your body permission to use its precious energy for the miracle of healing. Yes, sometimes we need to push through and take that step to strengthen ourselves. Like an athlete in training, action can restore strength and function, but even an elite athlete will follow up with rest and recovery. Rest is your friend.

Don't resent your body's need for it. Give yourself permission to passionately care for yourself. Embrace healing. Embrace rest. Honor your body while it works on your behalf.

With a heart of love for you!

Ronda

....

*"And he said, My presence shall go with you, and
I will give you rest,"* **Exod 33:14 (NASB).**

JOURNAL

What does rest look like for you today?

....
....
....
....
....
....
....
....
....
....
....
....
....
....
....
....
....
....
....

MY GREAT REWARD

Dear Susan,

You seek healing. You are doing all the things you know to do. You've turned your life upside down, hoping to regain what was lost, and healing will be your reward.

My dear friend, healing is a worthy quest, but there is a reward far greater than anything you could ever possess, and it cannot be taken away.

As I have passionately sought healing, it has bid to become the goal, the ultimate reward. Yet, every time I gained relief, it was never quite enough.

Health is a gift to be tenderly held and cherished. It allows us to reach, walk, give, and play. It offers many luxuries we often take for granted. Your health is worth pursuing and protecting, and our bodies are miraculously designed to heal.

Yes, our health is an invaluable resource in our daily lives and for good in this world. Seek it, walk in it, and enjoy it – all the while realizing if you see it as the ultimate pursuit, it will both consume and elude you.

I have sought health with the passion of a mother caring for her babies. Nothing drove me more. But in my passion and drive, I realized that my health, strength, and the ability to do things for my family is not the ultimate reward of my soul.

Over and over again, I have found that God is my reward, the treasure I seek. He is the strength of my heart and the love I desire. He is the provision I need, and the One who holds me and my precious family in His goodness, love, and care.

On this journey, I have gained a measure of health for which I am profoundly grateful. It is a priceless gift. However, I have also come to experience God as my shield, my comfort, my guide, my refuge, my strength, my provider, and yes, my exceedingly great reward.

With a heart of love for you!

Ronda

....

"Do not be afraid . . . I am your shield, your very great reward," **Gen 15:1 (NIV).**

JOURNAL

What do you seek as your reward?

....
....
....
....
....
....
....
....
....
....
....
....
....
....
....
....
....
....
....
....

ANOTHER SETBACK

Dear Susan,

Another setback. Yes, another bad report. A prognosis you did not want to hear or news that is completely shocking. I am sorry. As I write this, I am shedding tears with you. I imagine myself giving you a hug, and this letter is just my way of sitting with you.

Setbacks are painful to digest, and they can rob us of hope. HOPE. I love that word. It is full of life and the promise of life. It is what gets me out of bed most mornings.

HOPE . . . the promise that there is goodness and abundance NOW, in the moment of pain and setback, as well as the days ahead.

HOPE . . . the promise that there is more than what our physical eyes can see.

HOPE . . . the knowing that this setback does not mean YOU have been abandoned or forgotten. You are not alone.

No, you are NEVER alone. You are always connected to God . . . even when He feels a million miles away, and your heart doesn't feel it. The fact that you are in the middle of this setback does not mean you are alone or forgotten. No, it means the exact opposite. Pain confirms that you bear the image of God. God's response to brokenness is pain, and as His image-bearer, it is yours as well. You hurt deeply, but you don't hurt alone. HE hurts WITH you. Yes, my dear friend, He feels it all and holds you in the middle of your pain.

Even though you are experiencing a setback, there is HOPE. Dwell in HOPE with each thought and spoken word. There is always HOPE.

With a heart of love for you!

Ronda

....

"'The Lord is my portion,' says my soul, Therefore I have hope in Him," **Lam 3:24 (NASB).**

....

". . . for He has said, 'I WILL NEVER (under any circumstances) DESERT YOU (nor give you up nor leave you without support, nor will I in any degree leave you helpless), NOR WILL I FORSAKE or LET YOU DOWN or RELAX MY HOLD ON YOU (assuredly not),'" **Heb 13:5 (AMP).**

JOURNAL

As you face this setback, what words and thoughts of HOPE remind your heart that you are not alone?

....
....
....
....
....
....
....
....
....
....
....
....
....
....
....
....
....
....
....
....

THE POWER OF CHOICE

Dear Susan,

Everywhere you look there are "shoulds". Advice comes from healthcare professionals, family, friends, and other countless resources. You hear, "Do this; don't do that." It is a well-meaning list of "should" and "should nots" from people who care.

The external noise blares. So many voices and conflicting opinions leave you confused and anxious. Who is right? Who is wrong? You only want to know the things that will get you back on your feet. But how can you tell which caring *should* will do the trick?

At the same time, the chatter of internal noise competes. You fear the unknown and imagine a variety of possible scenarios. Your mind races. You just want to find the one *should* to make it all go away. As you pull the covers over your head, your heart wishes and cries for someone to fix you.

In our society, the task of healing typically starts with or belongs to our doctor or medical team. We trust them with the diagnosis, prognosis, and plan of action. We hope they can offer options to restore us, give us a few more days, or navigate the diagnosis for the best quality of life. We often see it as "their" job.

Medical professionals have a huge body of knowledge to share; they are an amazing resource. The problem with this scenario is often, in our vulnerable state, we relinquish our power, our choices, and our voice. These men and women seem to know the way, so we take a back seat and let them drive. They steer us on our road to resources and treatment choices. And we begin to act as though our healing is dependent on the right doctor, the right drug, the right access.

The maze of healthcare can leave us feeling powerless and voiceless. Because our bodies are weak, we have limited choices over our activities, relationships, and careers. Now, we are faced with limited choices over what our body endures, but we will do anything to get well, so we comply and move ahead.

Dear friend, hear me on this. You always have the power of choice. At times, the external noise grows loud, and the doctor's prognosis looms like the power of life or death. Our voice can be drowned out by fear, and we can no longer hear what our heart knows.

Stop for a minute. Breathe. In the quiet, take the time to listen. What does your heart hear, know, and want? Sometimes we focus so heavily on the *shoulds* and the experts, we don't stop and listen to the still small voice inside.

Please don't ignore medical advice. Absolutely, listen to every expert opinion. As you listen, do so from the perspective of choice. Take back the power to make loving decisions for yourself. Give your inner voice permission to tell the professionals what you need and to ask all your questions. You are the one living with the consequences of these decisions, so be empowered to ask questions, express your needs, and to choose.

Here's the truth. When we make decisions according to *shoulds*, we typically operate from a victim stance of fear and powerlessness. When we choose a course of action, we take our power back. Even when the decision is difficult, or there is one we don't want to make, we become participants in the recovery process. Healing isn't something that is done to us. We embrace and engage in the miracle. We shift from being reactionary victims of fear to being present recipients of healing. We reclaim power, choice, and love for ourselves.

Friend, move away from fear-based *shoulds*. Set them aside. What does your heart hear, know, and want? You are brave. You are courageous. You are strong. Embrace your course with power and love.

With a heart of love for you!

Ronda

....

"For God did not give us a spirit of timidity or cowardice or fear, but (He has given us a spirit) of power and of love and of sound judgment. . .,"
2 Tim 1:7a (AMP).

JOURNAL

What does your heart hear, know, and want?

....
....
....
....
....
....
....
....
....
....
....
....
....
....
....
....
....
....
....

THE STING OF TERMINAL

Dear Susan,

The word terminal stings. It cuts deep into our core eliciting fear and hopelessness. Webster's Dictionary defines terminal as *"occurring at or constituting the end of a series, concluding."* Yes, it is a dreaded word full of uncertainty and cruel finality.

We prefer to live avoiding and pretending this reality doesn't exist. Our mortality stirs up raw emotion; we fear the unknown and the loss of what we hold dear. We think it must apply to others, and we hope and pray it is never associated with our name. Though, in fact, aren't we all terminal?

Our lives go through many seasons that inevitably come to an end. Change is unavoidable. Without the acceptance of this reality, we can get stuck in a life we pretend will not end, a groundhog day of sorts.

Accepting that our current beautiful season is fleeting opens our eyes to see its rarity and all the gifts it brings. We can savor it like our favorite dessert served only on special holidays. Recognizing the rarity, and knowing it will end, brings delight and the ability to appreciate each breath in the moment.

Dear friend, we all live terminally. We have been given one physical body that will expire. However, YOU will never expire. The true you will never conclude. You will go on in the hearts and minds of those you love, and you will forever remain in the safe embrace of your Creator, the One who holds you and all eternity in His hands.

Maybe part of our dissonance with this word points to a greater, deeper understanding of our hearts: we will never be extinguished. We are living souls whose future is safe and destiny secure – life everlasting. Death is only a shadow. It has no sting because death is swallowed up in life. We have the sweet assurance that our lives will never end.

With a heart of love for you!

Ronda

....

"Even though I walk through the valley of the shadow of death I fear no evil, for You are with me; Your rod and Your staff they comfort me," **Ps 23:4 (NASB).**

....

"And when this perishable puts on the imperishable, and this mortal puts on immortality, then the Scripture will be fulfilled that says, 'Death is swallowed up in victory (vanquished forever). O Death, where is your victory? O Death, where is your sting?'" **I Cor 15:54-55 (AMP).**

JOURNAL

How would your days change if you lived
with the understanding that we are all
terminal?

....

....

....

....

....

....

....

....

....

....

....

....

....

....

....

....

....

....

IN THE WAITING

Dear Susan,

Today, your mind struggles to understand what has brought you to this moment, and you also wonder why the nightmare continues. Is this a cruel joke? When will it end? When will you find relief, either in heaven's arms or a body that is well and able?

You are exhausted. Oh, so tired of being in this in-between place with no fast-forward button to take you to the end. How do you navigate the messy middle of your story, this place of waiting, as well as the unknown?

It is hard to see clearly in the pain of waiting when the agony is relentless. You wait for healing, wait for answers, wait for treatment, or wait for heaven's welcome. My mom always said, "Waiting is the longest word in the Bible because we don't know when it will end."

You, my dear friend, are waiting for all you have hoped. Yes, your heart waits to know how it will all play out. It feels as though if you could know, control, or predict, it would somehow ease your heart and mind.

Susan, life is not meant to be experienced more than one moment at a time. I know your eyes are on the goal, but there is great purpose in the now. There is meaningful life to live in this moment. Please, don't miss it because you are only able to think about the thing for which your heart longs. You are exactly where you are meant to be. Let me assure you. You are not behind or ahead of schedule. You are in the perfect now.

You are fully alive with a beating heart, and this now will never come again. Live it fully. You are so brave and courageous. With eyes of faith, know there is purpose, love, and life that matters in the waiting. You are not abandoned and alone as you hang on expectantly. You are being held, and God is at work on your behalf – always.

Take heart, my friend. Don't stop living in the waiting. You are closer than you think.

With a heart of love for you!

Ronda

"*Our soul waits for the Lord; He is our help and our shield,*" **Ps 33:20 (NASB).**

"*Wait for the Lord; Be strong and let your heart take courage; Yes, wait for the Lord,*" **Ps 27:14 (NASB).**

JOURNAL

What would it look like to live fully in
the waiting?

....

....

....

....

....

....

....

....

....

....

....

....

....

....

....

....

....

....

....

....

....

....

YOU MATTER

Dear Susan

I am thinking about you. As I write this, I pray for you. Yes, you!

As a counselor, I enjoy individual time with people rather than being in large groups. I prefer sitting one-to-one, focused on seeing and hearing the other person. Today, I write with you in mind. You matter. I pray these words find their way into your hands and heart. It will be worth every hour of writing if you understand that YOU matter. Yes, you are important.

Illness can leave you feeling irrelevant, unimportant, and disregarded. But regardless of your strength or health, you hold the same worth and value as you did when you walked through this world prior to your illness. Strength and productivity do not define your value. Your ability to achieve and your worth are not the same thing. Even in the midst of your illness, the true you remains, and your significance is unshakeable. The way you live might be different right now, but you — the real you — has not changed, and never will. It's not about what you do or can't do. As long as you have breath, your presence and your thoughts matter in this world. You have beautiful, innate God-given value just being you. You were created in His very image.

Dear friend, may your heart understand and embrace how much you matter.

With a heart of love for you!

Ronda

....

"Then God said, 'Let Us make man in Our image, according to Our likeness… God created man in His own image, in the image of God He created him; male and female He created them,'" **Gen 1:26-27 (NASB).**

JOURNAL

Where do you find your sense of worth and value?

....

....

....

....

....

....

....

....

....

....

....

....

....

....

....

....

....

....

....

YOUR BODY IS FOR YOU

Dear Susan,

You may be feeling as though your body has let you down. It is not responding the way you had hoped. It isn't healing fast enough or not at all. There are days when it seems your healing road will never end.

Oh, dear friend, I hear you. I have felt the sting of discouragement when my body did not heal as I expected. It was a painful blow. As my days of treatment turned into months and years, I was left with a deep sense of shame and embarrassment as I wondered if my body was somehow defective. Why wasn't I healing?

I had always enjoyed good health and had taken for granted the miracle of thriving that happened in my body every day. I had expected to complete the treatment protocols and be back in the flow of my normal life. When that wasn't my reality, I was confused, disappointed, angry, and very scared. I had invested all my energy and resources into healing, and yet, I didn't see the fruit of my labors. In my dismay, I felt my body had betrayed me.

Over time, my anger softened, and my heart began to feel empathy. I realized how I had taken advantage of my health and harshly pushed my body as a servant doing my bidding. For the first time, I saw the abuses it had endured, and as I wept, I also began to hear the cries of my body. Gradually, my heart felt compassion for this earthly frame that had thanklessly served me. Year after year, it had quietly fought hard on my behalf in a million ways I did not see or know. It was <u>for</u> me, not against me. No, it wasn't betraying me. My body was desperately trying to protect me and bear the burden of my illness.

I grew to see my body as my ally. I embraced it as a cherished and trusted friend worth hearing, loving, and thanking. My healing journey was no longer about making demands or fighting. It was a path of patiently supporting and lovingly caring for myself through all the ups and downs.

My dear friend, your body fights for you, too. It is designed to look out for you. Yes, it is trying to do the very best for you. Love it. Thank it. Sit with it. Allow the awareness of your body to connect you to it with compassion. Touch your face and hands. Your body is a beautiful masterpiece created in the likeness of God. Even when it hurts, it is not betraying you. Give your body empathy, patience, and grace. It fights for you.

I know our relationship with our bodies can be complicated. If it has been abused, don't hate it. Don't reject it. It was not the perpetrator. If you abused it in some way, apologize and release regret. Forgive yourself. Honor your body as it honors you.

Give your body forgiveness for not being perfect and for being mortal. But also, delight in its miraculous power and ability to heal. Picture it healed. Speak wholeness over your body. Our thoughts and words are incredibly powerful. Your body prepares and responds as if your thoughts are reality. Caring for your body with loving thoughts and words can be a catalyst for wellness. Even if your body does not completely heal, your spirit can abide and rest in a place of compassion, safety, and love.

Your body is a gift, uniquely yours. It is working on your behalf. Give it love. Give it grace. Your body is ready to be embraced.

With a heart of love for you!

Ronda

....

"My frame was not hidden from You, When I was made in secret, and intricately and skillfully formed (as if embroidered with many colors) in the depths of the earth," **Ps 139: 15 (AMP).**

JOURNAL

Take some time to reflect and write about your relationship with your amazing body.

....

....

....

....

....

....

....

....

....

....

....

....

....

....

....

....

....

....

WHAT DOES THE WORD "SURRENDER" MEAN TO YOU?

Dear Susan,

Everything inside of you is objecting. This is not the way it is supposed to be.

Oh, friend! I hear the cry of your heart. It can be disorienting, scary, sad, and so very painful when life isn't turning out the way you had planned.

I dealt with illness for years and did everything in my power to get well. I traveled far for specialized treatments, spent money out of pocket, modified my diet, consulted with specialists, and took recommended supplements and medications. Finally, I gained a level of functional wellness; I cherished the level of normalcy I felt.

Then, out of nowhere, a new illness disabled me beyond anything I had experienced. It felt like someone pulled a chair out from under me.

I no longer had the freedom to come and go. Isolated in a prison of physical and emotional pain, any hope of regaining my former state of wellness seemed out of reach. This was my new life for the unforeseeable future. Fear, sadness, and anger overwhelmed me.

How could this have happened? Looking for answers and relief, I met with a doctor who told me, "Ronda, accept what comes." His words haunted me, and they made me angry!

Really??? Just accept this as my new lot in life? No! I won't!!!

With a family in my care, how could I accept this as my new normal? In my mind, acceptance or surrender meant giving in or losing. I wouldn't let this thing win! No way!! I must beat it. I must conquer.

Or, must I?

In my quiet moments, I felt conflicted, and my mind was filled with questions. *Is voicing my desire to be well in opposition to surrender? Is surrender about resigning myself to a designed path set for me? If so, should I continue to pray for healing? What does it mean if healing doesn't come?* With so many questions, my soul could not find rest.

However, what I came to understand about this word, "surrender," did bring rest.

Three truths brought clarity and gave me a new relationship with the word surrender:

1. Surrender is a process. It means affirming the reality of the situation, mourning the loss, and moving toward healing. Surrender doesn't take my voice. It gives my body a voice by allowing its reality to be heard.

2. Surrender releases my need to control. Holding tightly to what I cannot dictate leads to anxiety, fear, and torment. It forfeits peace and robs me of joy. Clinging to control leaves me bound to the craziness of the "what-ifs". It clouds my understanding, not allowing me to see and accept responsibility for what I can influence.

3. Surrender grounds me in this moment and opens me up to the possibilities of healing in the presence of love and grace. Fight and fear are guarded and lock me down in a dark bunker. They block out the light of truth that Love wants to reveal in my new reality.

As I sat with these revelations, I began to ask a new question. *What if surrender is not this thing I feared? Instead...*

- What if surrender is about having eyes to see?
- What if surrender allows us to wipe the fog from our pain-laden glasses allowing us to see our reality in a new way?
- What if surrender is about accepting the moment and being present in it, so we can experience God's comfort as He holds us in the middle of the tragedy?
- What if surrender is not holding things so tightly that they consume us, so we can no longer enjoy them? It's as if we're so concerned about losing the lollipop, we forget to taste it, enjoy it, and take it in.
- What if surrender offers a way to empty our burdens rather than empty our souls, thoughts, ideas, and dreams?
- What if surrender allows us to re-invent and grow within the reality of loss rather than allowing the loss to rob us and leave us hopeless?

- What if surrender is about living free of worries and outcomes we can't control, rather than "giving in" and relinquishing our power?

- What if surrender is about embracing the moment, in all its imperfections, so our hearts can know what it means to be fully alive?

- What if surrender is about accepting what I cannot change and allowing something new to be created?

- What if surrender allows us to rest by putting our body in a state of calm and peace where healing can enter and do its miraculous work?

- What if surrender is not saying "Yes" to illness but rather affirming that there is the need and the space to heal?

- What if surrender is not about "what should be," but seeds of strength that allow us to embrace our days as a gift?

- What if surrender is not being a victim to a designated plan but being available to dream anew and follow the path that God forges with us in the dark?

My sweet friend, I pray that as you acknowledge your new reality and grieve your loss, you will also find freedom, peace, and strength in the arms of surrender.

With a heart of love for you!

Ronda

"I am weary with my sighing; Every night I make my bed swim, I dissolve my couch with my tears. My eye has wasted away with grief . . . For the Lord has heard the voice of my weeping. The Lord has heard my supplication, The Lord receives my prayer," **Ps 6:6-9 (NASB).**

JOURNAL

What does the word "surrender" mean to you?

....

....

....

....

....

....

....

....

....

....

....

....

....

....

....

....

....

....

....

....

TRYING TO GET "HER" BACK

Dear Susan,

Illness can leave you feeling as though you have lost yourself. Often, it changes your body, your abilities, your perspective, and your experience of life. You may look in the mirror and not recognize the person staring back at you, making you wonder where you have gone. Your heart worries that you don't exist anymore.

You seek medical advice, health gurus, and follow all the latest and greatest tips to get her back. But you fear you have lost her forever. You feel indefinitely scarred or altered. Months and years have gone. . . eroding the person you once knew. You fear never seeing her again. Oh, the tears fall.

My dear friend, please hear me. You don't have to wait to get back to the former version of yourself. You needn't be completely healed to see her again. You are here, and you are still YOU. In this moment, you are not less than or inferior to your past or future self. You are preserved. No, you don't have to wait to be someone in the future, nor do you need to reach back to a past version of yourself. The yesterday you is not gone. The true you can never be lost.

I lived many years waiting to get back to a version of my former self. I felt so very lost. I spent years trying to recover what I believed to be my glory days of health, confident that in the process I would also recover myself. However, the girl from those glory days was the very same woman who endured, persevered, and trusted the path that was forged in the dark. Parts of me shined brighter in the darkness while other parts were harder to see. But my laughter, love, desires, joys, and all that made me truly me remained the same.

Oh, weary friend, listen to these words of truth.

"The Lord is your keeper: the Lord is the shade upon your right hand. The sun will not smite you by day, nor the moon by night. The Lord will preserve you from all evil: he will preserve your soul. The Lord will preserve your going out and your coming in from this time forth and always," **Ps 121:5-8 (NKJV).**

Listen to the Psalmist. God has preserved you. Your body may change, your mind covered in fog. Your emotions may cry out, but He preserves you always. The actions and words of others may change, and you may feel different, but it doesn't alter <u>you</u>. Your perspective may blur, but you, He has preserved.

Illness and injury cannot rob you of you. Susan is still Susan, growing in wisdom, empathy, understanding, strength, patience, and love. You are an oak rooted and grounded in God's love. You cannot be cut down. Your roots grow deeper, and you become more you. You remain loved, cherished, and preserved.

With a heart of love for <u>you</u>!

Ronda

....

"You are the Lord, You alone. You have made heaven, the heaven of heavens, with all their host, the earth and all that is on it, the seas and all that is in them; and You preserve all of them; and the host of heaven worships you," **Neh 9:6 (ESV).**

JOURNAL

What truths, activities, items, or people remind your heart that you have not been lost?

....

....

....

....

....

....

....

....

....

....

....

....

....

....

....

....

....

....

THERE IS GOOD

Dear Susan,

I am writing this letter as I celebrate the birthday of a dear loved one in heaven. It is a sad day full of reflection, a bag of mixed emotions. My relationship with this loved one was complicated. Though often painful, there was also good.

I have come to realize that most things are neither all good nor all bad, and it is important to acknowledge it all if we want to walk in the truth of our full story and be free to heal.

What do you face today? It may not be good. You may not feel well. If so, I am truly sorry. Let yourself see the pain, the sadness. Let yourself feel it. You don't have to feel it alone. Talk to a trusted friend or professional counselor; journal; tell God all about it. Let the tears flow, my sweet friend.

Once you sit with the painful truth, I challenge you to keep looking for the good. It may be wrapped in unexpected packages or difficult to see at first glance, but keep looking and expect it. Good is always there because God is always present. He is the good.

I am learning that evil is overcome in anticipating, finding, and seeing the good. Not that our circumstances change; often, they do not, but we can go higher. Look for the good in the past, in the moment, and the future. When we focus on the good, we experience its gifts. We discover peace, rest, joy, and gratitude. It opens our eyes to love. Of course, it does, because He is the source of all that is good, and He overcomes.

Remember, in the middle of pain, good doesn't subject itself to evil's demands. It doesn't pay evil's price or ruminate to find an equal blow or hold it in a headlock to punish. No, good rises above. It loves, it forgives, it releases. It goes higher, and yes, it overcomes.

So, as I sit with sadness today, I will acknowledge the bad and the painful, but I will also look for good because it was there, and it is here, and it will guide me into my future. Good does overcome.

With a heart of love for you!

Ronda

....

"Surely goodness and mercy will follow me all the days of my life, and I will live in the house of the Lord forever," **Ps 23:6 (NASB).**

....

"Do not be overcome and conquered by evil, but overcome evil with good," **Rom 12:21 (AMP).**

JOURNAL

Where do you see good in the middle of your story?

....
....
....
....
....
....
....
....
....
....
....
....
....
....
....
....
....
....
....
....
....

THE OPPORTUNITY OF VULNERABILITY

Dear Susan,

Today, you feel completely stripped down. As you look around, the losses are too numerous to count. You see yourself nakedly bare, and you feel vulnerable. Just reading the word vulnerable leaves you uncomfortable and raw.

You have spent your days shoring up everything around you to construct a life of safety, security, certainty, and control. Now in one fatal swoop, the legs of the chair have been knocked out from under you, and you feel vulnerable.

Vulnerability is a place of being open and susceptible. Being so exposed carries a terrifying ring, and oh, how we want to run from it. You didn't choose to be in this state, and you are scared. It may also tap into some of your worst fears by reaching into your childhood and echoing deep hurts and betrayals you've encountered along the way. The thought of being vulnerable can be unsettling on many levels, shaking you to your very core.

Oh, dear friend, could it be that the vulnerability and openness you most fear also ushers in an opportunity? Yes, an unexpected opportunity to dig deep, opening you to see, try, and experience things anew? Vulnerability can fuel the desire to learn, change, and trust. It opens a door deep into your soul. This, my dear friend, is the place of change and exponential growth. It reveals the things that have kept you stuck or on autopilot, and in this tender place, healing is possible from the inside out.

Do you see it? When your inner being is vulnerable, open, and permeable, life-giving newness can enter. Embrace your vulnerability. See life through the eyes of your child-like heart. Take in the wonder of it all like you have never experienced or may have forgotten.

Dear friend, your vulnerability is beautiful and oh, so precious. It is a gateway to the new that is waiting for you. In this sacred space, you are open and permeable to the powerful healing gifts of love and grace. Allow vulnerability to open your eyes and deepest longings. Love and grace will meet you here and bathe you in peace.

With a heart of love for you!

Ronda

....

*"Listen carefully, I am about to do a new th*ing, Now it will spring forth; Will you not be aware of it? I will even put a road in the wilderness, *Rivers in the desert,"* **Isa 43:19 (AMP).**

JOURNAL

In vulnerable moments, how can you
invite newness, love, healing, and con-
nection with God and others?

....
....
....
....
....
....
....
....
....
....
....
....
....
....
....
....
....
....

DEVELOPING CLEARER VISION

Dear Susan,

Your world is small. It feels as though the picture on the TV of your life has gone from a large screen with surround sound to a tiny picture playing in slow motion. There has been a huge shift, not only in how you live your life but every element of it. Not only has your sphere diminished, but you are also aware that your strength to maintain or engage is more limited.

Though your world may now be small, your vision doesn't have to be. From this place, you have the opportunity to see life's colors like never before. Yes, you heard me right. You are no longer twirling through life at the speed of light. Now, you have the perspective to see life with a new resolve from a fresh point of view. You can clearly see what truly matters and is most important to you. In the stillness, you now have an awareness that allows you to experience the simple and yet, beautiful moments of your life. You observe many things you once walked by without noticing, such as the individual petals of a flower, the softness of the towel you hold, and details of the faces you so love. Yes, from your vantage point, you see things you once missed. You, my friend, have been given vision.

How often do we fly through our day without truly seeing or tasting life? We mindlessly ignore the gifts presenting themselves and begging for our attention.

Several years ago, I was at a treatment facility, and I overheard others talking about a short path nearby that led to a beautiful creek. I set a goal for the week to walk the entire length of this path to see for myself the peaceful, flowing water I had painted in my mind. Determined, I set my sights.

One day, I evoked every ounce of strength I could muster and headed out on a quest to find the beautiful creek. When I made it, to my complete delight, it did not disappoint. It was absolutely breathtaking and refreshing for my soul.

On the way back, while basking in the achievement of my outing, I came upon a huge bush with the biggest and juiciest berries I had ever seen! Blackberries spilled off the bush in abundance, free for the taking. I was so excited and hungry! I began picking as many as my hands would hold, and then, it hit me. This blackberry bush was on the path as I walked to the creek. I just did not see it. My eyes were on the goal at the end of the path, and even though I was hungry, I had overlooked this huge bush and its delicious offerings! It made me wonder, *How often have I walked hastily through life with a goal in mind and missed out on the simple and yet, profound gifts that were mine for the taking?*

Dear friend, your days may be slow and small right now, but your days are precious. Look around with new vision. What do you see? Take it in. Savor it with awe. As you pause to look with eyes of gratitude, your vision will expand. You will begin to see the picture of your life in 3D. The beauty that has always been there will jump out at you. Don't walk by it anymore. Open your eyes and see.

With a heart of love for you!

Ronda

....

"They feast on the abundance of your house, and you give them drink from the river of your delights. For with you is the fountain of life; in your light do we see light," **Ps 36:8-9 (ESV).**

JOURNAL

What are the things you see, enjoy, and savor that you didn't notice or value before your illness?

....

....

....

....

....

....

....

....

....

....

....

....

....

....

....

....

....

DO YOU FEEL FORGOTTEN?

Dear Susan,

The crisis of your news has faded, and you are grateful the dust has settled. However, your phone is now silent, notes have slowed, the meal train has stopped, and visitors are few and far between. You find yourself navigating a new world where you feel shut away and unable to keep up. Life goes on, and you have a sense of being left behind. You feel forgotten.

Whether in a hospital, nursing home, psychiatric facility, or at home, the loneliness resonates deep inside, and questions ring loud. Does anyone care? Does anyone remember? Has even God forgotten me?

Pain has a way of making us feel abandoned. I know it has in my life. The feeling of being left behind by people I loved was so difficult, but it was even harder to grapple with wondering if God had forgotten me. Even though I have known God's incredible love for me for a long time, there have been moments of overwhelming pain when I couldn't always connect with it. At times, I even doubted His love existed, which created excruciating anguish all its own. I felt abandoned and yes, forgotten.

My friend, if you find yourself in that place today, let me assure you. If there is one thing of which you can be certain, it is this: God has not forgotten you. Please, hear me. He holds you forever in His love. Nothing can separate you from it. <u>Absolutely nothing</u>!

It just so happens; I was reminded of this beautiful truth today. My son recently graduated from high school and set out on new adventures. This morning, as I thought of him, a wave of tears and emotions hit me. Although I can't physically see and touch him, nothing can separate my son from my love. I will always hold him in my heart. It isn't possible for me to forget him. He is mine.

Do you see? If I, being an imperfect mother, can't forget, how much more will your Heavenly Father not remember? He created you. Every cell of your body is known by Him. His presence is affirmed in your every breath, and He says, "You are mine." He has not forgotten. It just isn't possible.

My dear friend, the God of the universe walks every day of this journey with you, and when the time comes, He will also walk you home. He could not and will not ever forget.

With a heart of love for you!

Ronda

....

"Can a woman forget her nursing child and have no compassion on the son of her womb? Even these may forget, but I will not forget you. Indeed, I have inscribed (a picture of) you on the palms of my hands," **Isa 49:15-16 (AMP).**

JOURNAL

Write about someone you could not forget, and then, reflect on God's knowing love and presence in your life.

....
....
....
....
....
....
....
....
....
....
....
....
....
....
....
....
....
....

THE STORY YOU TELL YOURSELF

Dear Susan,

What story are you telling yourself about the future? We all have a narrative running in our head, don't we? The movie can be based on our worst fears, or it can be filled with hopes and dreams. Which is it for you? Do you compose the worst possible outcomes, draining your strength and sabotaging your hope as they replay in your mind? After facing so much difficulty and pain, it can be hard not to expect or fear the worst of all possibilities.

Maybe you dare not venture into the unknown, and you avoid thinking about the future at all. Fear of pain, repeated disappointment, and loss are reminders that you just don't want to go there.

Oh, Susan, it can be excruciating to walk into the unknowns of the future, especially when the tomorrow of your mind leaves no room for hope. It is here that my heart longs to speak to you.

Expectations, possibilities, and hope are woven into the story you tell yourself, and they have a powerful influence on your emotional and physical health. Athletes are the perfect example of this very truth. They often visualize the event for which they train long before they compete. They see themselves crossing the finish line, scoring the goal, accomplishing what their heart desires long before the actual event. They see it, rehearse it, and expect it. They don't focus on anyone else's race but their own. Their body prepares as their mind and spirit rehearse with a unified sense of vision and hope.

Dear friend, this is your race. Your body will prepare for what you anticipate and visualize in your future. Your expectations, thoughts, and words hold so much power and potential. They affect the cells of your body. Your vision for the future leads the way to realize your heart's longings.

What story does your mind's eye write? You will have hard days when your vision and hope might be difficult to see, and that is okay. No matter your circumstances, there is hope, and there will be another day beyond what you see and feel today, whether it be here on earth or finally in your heavenly home. Your tomorrow is glorious beyond anything you could ask or even imagine. Your dreams may not yet be fulfilled, but hang on. They are as real as today, and there is a beautiful future waiting for you.

With a heart of love for you!

Ronda

....

"Now to Him who is able to do far more abundantly beyond all that we ask or think, according to the power that works within us," **Eph 3:20a (NASB).**

JOURNAL

What is the vision in your heart for the future?

....
....
....
....
....
....
....
....
....
....
....
....
....
....
....
....
....
....
....
....

I GET TO TAKE CARE OF ME

Dear Susan,

Self-care can become overwhelming. Your body may need many things to heal or rehabilitate. It can feel all-consuming and at times, like a full-time job. The very thought of self-care may also bring guilt and the thoughts, *I don't do enough, or I don't know where to start.* There are days when you want to pull the covers over your head and wish it all away. I hear you. For years, I did as well.

This morning, I woke up with a new insight that turned that thought on its head: *I get to take care of me today.* As I pondered that notion, I began to see caring for myself through a new lens of anticipation and pleasure instead of guilt and duty. It brought a smile to my face because I knew this perspective would challenge old beliefs and change how I care for myself.

I once held the belief that my needs are not important. I would not allow myself to need extra or be an inconvenience. I did not feel worthy of nurture or care. Can you relate? Well, that belief is bogus! The truth is each one of us is worthy of loving support and healing. You, my friend, are worth it, and taking care of your body will also serve to nourish and heal your soul, reminding you of your worthiness.

Yes, we get to show up and care for ourselves, and respond to our needs by doing things that make us healthy, happy, and whole. It's not a chore. We have the privilege of self-care. And in this nourishing space, we are present, attuned to our body, and ready to show up for the next nurturing practice or resource available to us.

With this perspective in mind, I took a walk today. As I noticed nature, I realized this concept of loving attention goes beyond us and has a powerful rippling effect. From this place of caring for ourselves, we learn to take care of the animals and the earth. This "get to" mindset of care benefits our environment as well as those for whom we care. Yes, nourishing ourselves makes us stronger for the world and those we love most, and we also model what self-care looks like to those little eyes watching our every move.

So, my friend, just as you are not a burden, self-care is not a chore, it is a delight. Your body is a gift, and you have been entrusted with this miraculous treasure. It is not to be used or abused as a servant. Your body is to be prioritized, respected, and loved. Don't care for it out of sheer duty or fear of disease, but as a vessel worthy of honor and love.

I woke up this morning with joy at the thought of taking care of me today. I want to capture this thought and feeling. I want to hold on to it, and never let it go. Will you join me?

With a heart of love for you!

Ronda

....

"I will give thanks to You, for I am fearfully and wonderfully made; Wonderful are Your works, And my soul knows it very well," **Ps 139:14-16 (NASB).**

JOURNAL

What beliefs keep you from enjoying the practice of caring for yourself?

....

....

....

....

....

....

....

....

....

....

....

....

....

....

....

....

....

....

....

GRATITUDE

Dear Susan,

Today, you are feeling the heaviness of all the burdens you carry. It is so much. Your mind can't even absorb it all, and you find yourself over-whelmed, anxious, or numb. You bear the weight of the unknown, the deep grief of loss, and the pain of illness as your body cries out. As you hold it all, there is desperation for relief, but you don't see an escape. You can't find an exit door. You are locked in a prison of pain. You peer out the barred window longing for a different view and a place of rest outside these gray walls. Your heart cries for release and to be free . . . if only for a moment

Dear friend, I have found a place of freedom with awe-inspiring views, and you can walk out the door and access it any time. It is a breathtaking overlook offering brilliance and wonder as far as the eyes can see. The name of this overlook, gratitude. There is no cost for admission, it is always available, and the sun is continually shining to reveal its gifts. Yes, it is there waiting for you.

It is a place to lay down burdens, gain a new perspective, and see the vast beauty that is already there. From this perch of gratitude, we witness and embrace the love and magnificence of our very Source of breath. We see the gifts, and our hearts sing, "It is good!" As our hearts swell, our souls are filled with a joy that flows in steady supply.

Each morning, I lay down my backpack of worries and cares, and give myself permission to wholeheartedly embrace gratitude . . . if only for a moment. I climb onto the railing of the overlook, peer off into the distance, and begin to count my gifts. As my gifts grow in number, I let go of the railing and open my arms wide. I glimpse the unending nature of His love, the beauty of His presence, and the Creator who is also mine. Unfettered, my heart rises in thankfulness, and it is a holy sanctuary of wonder and awe that frees me on the wings of joy . . . if only for a moment.

Friend, there is plenty of room at the overlook. Come, and set your heart free. You will fly.

With a heart of love for you!

Ronda

. . . .

"Give thanks to the Lord, for He is good. For His lovingkindness is everlasting," **Ps 136:1 (NASB).**

JOURNAL

Join me at the overlook by writing five things for which you are grateful in the space below.

....
....
....
....
....
....
....
....
....
....
....
....
....
....
....
....
....
....

LIVING A LIFE OF ABUNDANCE

Dear Susan,

Today, you may feel overwhelmed by all you seem to lack. There are demands and needs in your life, and you see a huge gap between the needs and what you possess. You can't help but feel there is not enough.

Dear friend, I know it can feel as though you are living on the edge of disaster. There have been times the demands of my life felt insurmountable, and I was utterly overwhelmed by my lack of resources, strength, and endurance. Once, I cared for my parents and children while also recovering from a complicated surgery. I had no idea how I would be able to do it. How would I provide for my own needs, not to mention those of my family, who depended on me in many ways? In this place of perceived lack, I realized there was a choice before me. *What if I live as though I have everything I need?* How would things change? What if I didn't worry about lack. Instead, what if I walked through each day knowing that my needs were already met?

I began watching with anticipation, and I opened my heart and arms to every avenue of provision. It was crazy how this simple question, "What if I lived as though I have everything I need?" changed my approach to life. This concept became a paradigm shift that lightened my burdens, relieved stress, and aided in my healing. It improved the sense of ease and joy in my life, and I worried a bit less.

Dear friend, don't judge this moment solely on loss or disappointment. Let yourself feel them. They are real. They are witnesses and expressions of your pain. But also know, in the midst of these moments of agonizing pain and grief, abundance is waiting and inviting you to embrace the gifts it offers, both seen and unseen.

What if you lived as though you have everything you need for today? Anticipating with eyes of faith can help you see provisions for each moment. I don't know what you need, but there is One who knows, and His love is deeper and greater than any pit of darkness. He knows. He cares. He provides — moment by moment. You may not see it all right now, but there is abundance for you.

With a heart of love for you!

Ronda

....

"Look at the birds of the air, that they do not sow, nor reap nor gather into barns, and yet your heavenly Father feeds them. Are you not worth much more than they?" **Matt 6:26 (NASB).**

....

"And God is able to make all grace abound to you, so that always having all sufficiency in every-thing, you may have an abundance for every good deed," **2 Cor 9:8 (NASB).**

JOURNAL

What if you lived as though you have everything you need?

....
....
....
....
....
....
....
....
....
....
....
....
....
....
....
....
....
....
....
....
....
....

HOPE, FAITH & LOVE

Dear Susan,

Today, you feel hopeless. You don't see the progress or healing for which you had strived. You wonder if your efforts even matter anymore. That for which you hoped, you do not see; instead, there are many unknowns. You wish for a guarantee. How can you live not knowing for sure? How can you move forward when you don't know what that next step will bring? How do you continue to hope for a better tomorrow when your eyes can only see the impossible?

Oh, my friend, I have asked myself those questions and many more. I had worked so hard and come so far, and yet, what I desired felt so far away. I knew hope gave me the strength to endure the pain and take steps forward. Yet, it felt so fleeting. I would feel hopeful for a moment and then something as simple as a phone call, a thought, or a word would bring me face-to-face with the unknown and rob me of this priceless commodity. Any hope could easily shift or disappear with the winds of disappointment, loss, or setbacks. I wondered how long I could keep going without a guarantee.

Finally, I began to feel grounded even though the earth was shaking under my feet. I realized if I based my hope on the threatening tremors of the unknown, I would never be able to enjoy the peace and strength that come with hope. No, I couldn't control the vibrations of my circumstances, but I could hear the music between the echoes of the vibrato, and I could choose the song to sing.

You see, hope is not secured by the guarantee of making the trembling stop. It is experienced in the midst of the rumblings as a sweet melody that is intricately connected to the mystery and certainty of faith and love. The three are a powerful trinity working in perfect harmony like a beautifully orchestrated symphony. Together, they feed and sustain the human soul. You can't experience the full beauty of hope without opening your heart to hear them all.

Faith is the vision and intention of our hearts that is not yet secured. This powerful force allows us to anticipate the mystery of what is not yet seen. The strength of love gives us the assurance it is safe to trust, provides a resting place for our soul, and secures the only guarantee that hope truly needs: the promise you are loved now and forever. As a result, hope is awakened and rises above our circumstances and the miry clay that wants to hold us down demanding a guarantee in order to release us.

You see, my friend, hope is not based on a temporal guarantee. It rides on the wings of faith and is deeply rooted and grounded in an eternal love that assures us our future is secure and there is so much beauty yet to see. May your heart awaken and sing the song of hope.

With a heart of love for you!

Ronda

....

"And now these three remain: faith, hope and love. But the greatest of these is love," **I Cor 13:13 (NIV).**

....

"Now faith is the assurance of things hoped for, the conviction of things not seen," **Heb 11:1 (NASB).**

JOURNAL

On what temporal guarantee do you base
your hope?

....
....
....
....
....
....
....
....
....
....
....
....
....
....
....
....
....
....

LONGING TO LIVE PAIN-FREE

Dear Susan,

You are in pain. How you wish you could be free of it. Pain is relentless, and the days can be brutal and endless. My heart hurts with you. I wrote the following reflection while also sitting with deep physical and emotional pain of my own. I had often assumed that if I followed all the rules and lived in a predictable way, I would lead a somewhat idyllic life of safety with foreseeable outcomes. However, that has not been my story. I have come face-to-face with the fact that we are all human, and we live in a world that experiences heartache and loss of which none are immune.

Yes, there are lives that appear charmed in our world of "smile for the camera," but the truth is none of us leave this world without sorrow. The experiences of both pain and pleasure are beautifully human. Dear friend, no matter your circumstance, my prayer is that you will find comfort, peace, and relief in this world of pain.

* * *

Pain-free. Isn't the absence of pain what we really want? We seek pleasure to lessen or mask the pain. We chase fame to lessen the pain of feeling inadequate, unworthy, unloved. We seek health to avoid the pain of sickness. We accumulate wealth to avoid the pain of want and hunger. We search for love to heal the pain of rejection. We welcome companionship and friendship to lessen the pain of being alone.

Pain is hard to avoid. Even when we desperately try, it follows us from childhood into adulthood. Pain shadows us as we live our lives through tragedy, disappointment, loss, betrayal, and sickness. We try to mask it, muffle it, numb it, but it is always there. Certain experiences make it louder, with an intensity so great we can hardly bear the noise of our hearts and body as they cry out. Other experiences make it more distant, less visceral so that we hardly hear the pain at all. We try to run, but the ache follows. We attempt to stamp it out, but it survives. We try to ignore or mute it, but it will not be silenced.

Oh, Pain, you are a companion on the road of life. We can either despise and curse you, or we can sit with you and listen to the pulse of your reality. Learn the lessons you teach. Breathe in the wisdom that comes from your presence. Look at the injustices and losses to which you point.

Yet, we long to be free of you. Yes, pain-free. I know I do. As I write these words, the tears flow. What would it be like? What would we be like?

If we didn't know pain, we would not be able to connect with the human experience. We would not have empathy, compassion, love. Pain connects us; it unifies us. It drives us to heal, change, justice, courage, faith, and love. Pain challenges us to rise above, to believe, to hope, to endure, and to grow.

Yes, pain makes us strong, and yet, we often see it as a sign of weakness, because it makes us feel vulnerable, out of control, broken, frustrated, angry. We view it as an enemy, a presence that wants to steal our joy and extinguish our life. We experience pain as a place of being alone, unsafe, or punished.

Yet, pain does not mean we are alone, forgotten, abandoned, unloved, or punished. In the middle of pain, we are still held by the One who knows our name, hears our cries, holds us tenderly, and feels our every pain.

What if we were to consider pain a friend rather than a foe? Is that possible? Could we see it as a life-giving force as pain gives way to life in childbirth, or gives way to the life to come when we take our last breath? Could we see it as a companion whose goal is to free us rather than consume us? A force of life that moves us from what was to what could be. A friend that alerts us to danger and the need for attention or intervention.

Could pain be a process of healing and restoration, a process of life? Without pain, we would not learn. We would not strive. We would not rest. We would not grow. We would not heal.

Okay, Pain, may your presence be a reminder of all that we have gained rather than all we have lost. A reminder of our humanity and the process of healing that connects our heart to others. A reminder of our complete dependence and need for our Creator. The One who sustains, loves, comforts, and provides for us as we walk through this world of pain.

* * *

My dear friend, may you rise to greater heights and know a deeper love as you move through this journey with pain.

With a heart of love for you!

Ronda

....

"Though the fig tree should not blossom And there be no fruit on the vines, Though the yield of the olive should fail And the fields produce no food, Though the flocks should be cut off from the fold and there be no cattle in the stalls, Yet I will exult in the LORD, I will rejoice in the God of my salvation. The Lord GOD is my strength, And He has made me feet like hinds' feet, And makes me walk on my high places," **Hab 3:17-19 (NASB)**.

JOURNAL

Take time to write about your journey
with pain.

....
....
....
....
....
....
....
....
....
....
....
....
....
....
....
....
....
....
....

LEARNING TO SOAR

Dear Susan,

There are many times you wonder how you will make it through the day. Where will you find the endurance to get from point A to point B? The normal and even simple demands of the day become overwhelming tasks that take all of your strength. Oh, friend, I hear you. It is difficult when there is so much you want to do, and yet, you can't predict the energy or stamina your body will have from one moment to the next.

Years ago, before the days of delivery, I was physically unable to go to the grocery store for food and other essentials, so a friend shopped for me. (I have such wonderful friends!) However, time constraints made it impossible for her to bring the groceries to my home. We chose a convenient meeting place near the local interstate. In my weak state, I had only driven my car a few times since returning from my lengthy stay at a treatment center. I could drive safely, but the idea of navigating the busy interstate in my bustling city overwhelmed me.

As I left my neighborhood, I said to God, "My brain is foggy, and my body feels weak. I need a back road to get to my destination. Please show me where to go!"

I felt a gentle nudging to take an immediate right turn. I thought, "I must have heard wrong, this is crazy, I can't get there by turning that direction."

But I was learning to trust those promptings, so I turned right. Immediately, I looked up and saw a beautiful eagle soaring above me. It was flying low, and I was amazed at its wingspan. It was completely breathtaking.

I said out loud, "Is that an eagle?" I started to argue with myself. That can't be an eagle. We don't have eagles around here." It was as if God said, "Go with it, Ronda. Trust Me on this one. It's an eagle!"

Then, the arguing stopped, and a familiar verse came to my mind.

> *But those who hope in the Lord will renew their strength. They will soar on wings as eagles, they shall run and not grow weary, they shall walk and not be faint,* **Isa 40:31 (NIV).**

New words spoke clearly to my heart. "Complete trust and dependence on God for each moment of my day, even making this right turn. This is what it means to soar."

I was soaring. I started to cry! I had always wondered what this verse in Isaiah really meant. I hadn't known how it would manifest in my life. Now, my heart understood. I just needed to spread my wings and stop trying to make sense of it all, stop trying to control the future, but rather to be in the now and just let God carry me.

As these thoughts filled my mind, through the tears, I noticed a new street that had opened while I was out of town. I turned onto the new road and discovered it was the back way that led to my destination. The crazy right turn was not so crazy after all. Yes, God had been carrying me.

Since that day, when I leave my house, I look up with new eyes and inevitably, I will see a hawk or a bird soaring above. The prompting comes to my heart, "Ronda, just spread your wings and soar."

It is a beautiful and gentle reminder to not run in my own strength. When I allow myself to be in the moment with God and let Him carry my worries, I soar.

My sweet friend, today, will you join me? Instead of looking at all that needs to be done, look up and see the reminders, accept the urge to fly, just spread your wings and soar.

With a heart of love for you!

Ronda

P.S. A few weeks later, I heard neighbors talking about an eagle's nest they had discovered nearby. The news brought a knowing smile. It was an eagle!

....

"Even to your old age, I shall be the same, And even to your graying years I shall bear you! I have done it, and I shall carry you; And I shall bear you, and I shall deliver you." **Isa 46:4 (NASB).**

JOURNAL

What does "accepting the urge to fly" mean to you?

....

....

....

....

....

....

....

....

....

....

....

....

....

....

....

....

....

....

....

LET'S KEEP IN TOUCH

Dear Friend,

We have come to the end of the letters to Susan. Thank you for taking this journey through joy, pain, grief, and beauty with me. It has been my honor to walk with you. There are no easy answers, reasons, or formulas that make it okay. It is not okay, and I am sorry you are suffering. My prayer is that through these pages, you have found a measure of comfort that will help you process grief, pain, and loss so that you may live with a little more joy, hope, and peace.

I know your path continues, but you don't have to do it alone. If you enjoyed these letters and would like a community of support and additional resources, I am here for you. As one who walks my own healing road and has had many years of experience as a counselor, I mentor women who are navigating the painful and confusing waters of illness. I have created a unique online community, as well as other resources, that will support and help you experience a meaningful life of hope and beauty as you walk out your story. I welcome you to join us and would love to keep in touch.

Many blessings on your healing journey!

With a heart of love for you!

Ronda

P.S. You can learn more about the community and additional resources at rondabarney.com. Can't wait to see you there!

IN MEMORIAM OF
SUSAN C. NEIBEL

1958-2020

This book is offered in loving memory of Susan C. Neibel. How do you capture in words a soul who was bigger than life? Susan had a profound impact on me, and I know there are many who could testify of the influence she had on them as well. As one in the chorus, I am profoundly grateful for the opportunity to glimpse her beautiful heart and to witness the love and compassion she had for her family, friends, community, and the world. She was an incredible woman who lived her life with passion and exhibited a courageous and contagious love for God and others.

Susan truly saw people, and she touched them with an indelible mark of love and grace. I am one of those individuals. During her last days, with limited strength, she continued to love boldly. I am eternally grateful for the privilege to have known this extraordinary woman; to witness her passion, love, and creativity; and to hear her heart's reflections as she neared her heavenly home.

She was a spiritual sister who knew the crucible of suffering, and yet, she lived embracing a greater hope. My desire to somehow offer her a small measure of comfort was graciously received but also eclipsed, as I was the one most encouraged, inspired, and changed by our interactions. Everywhere she went, Susan impacted people's lives with her love and example, and even in her last days, from the isolation of her bed, she poured into mine. Susan was a bright light in this world. May her light continue to shine through her legacy and memory. Her kindnesses, generous spirit, and love will never be forgotten.

Ronda Barney

THANK YOU LETTER

Dear Autumn,

Without your introduction to Susan, the letters in this book would likely remain in my journal, and the dream of sending them into the world would not have become a reality. With all my heart, I thank you. Thank you for introducing me to Susan and orchestrating this incredible journey. Your suggestion that the three of us share a group email as I sent the letters to Susan was brilliant. It gave our hearts a place to reflect, laugh, support, cry, pray, and love together. It was a time that forged a beautiful friendship between us for which I will forever be grateful. You often said the exchange of the letters was a sacred space, and I wholeheartedly agree. Thank you for initiating and engaging in that space with us. I felt the Hand of grace and love holding the three of us as we corresponded during Susan's last months and days. What a privilege to have shared that experience with you. It was truly life changing. You have continued to support me as I have taken steps to publish this book and share these letters with the world. I could not be more grateful for your encouragement and listening ear. I love you, my friend.

Love,

Ronda

ABOUT THE AUTHOR

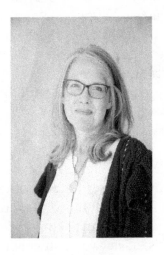

Ronda Barney, LCSW, RD is a mentor to women facing life-changing illness. Through writing, speaking, and mentoring, she helps women experiencing the complexities of illness give voice to their pain, awaken to hope, and experience their hearts fully alive.

Ronda practiced as a Registered Dietitian at Georgetown University Hospital and George Washington University Hospital in Washington, D.C. She also worked for fourteen years as an outpatient clinical therapist and dietitian with Meier Clinics in Fairfax, Va. She has been a featured conference speaker and appears on podcasts sharing her message of hope and resilience. She is also the creator of several online resources and a mentoring program, devoted to helping women facing illness find the freedom and strength to live their unique, beautiful life, fully alive.

As a new mom, and while practicing as a clinical psychotherapist and dietitian, Ronda found herself as a patient, trying to navigate the unknowns and anguish of a complex and life-changing illness. Even with her education and mental health background, she was not prepared for the emotional and physical toll a devastating illness can have on one's life. Through years of illness and recovery, Ronda began to give voice to her pain, and she found paths, like roads in the desert, to hope, joy, peace, and purpose. She is passionate about helping others articulate their own pain and find these same paths, even in the midst of loss and the unknown. Ronda and her husband, Chris, have two adult children and live in Dallas, Texas.

You can connect with her, and learn more about additional resources at rondabarney.com.